The Quick and Easy Guide to Healing Herbs

Dr. Susan's Healthy Living
drsusanshealthyliving.com

I0417221

Facebook.com/DrSusanRichards
drsusanshealthyliving@gmail.com
(650) 561-9978

Mention of specific companies or products in this book does not suggest endorsement by the author or publisher. Internet addresses and telephone numbers for resources provided in this book were accurate at the time it went to press.

ISBN 978-1512155716

Note

The information in this book is meant to complement the advice and guidance of your physician, not replace it. It is very important that any person who has medical problems be evaluated by a physician. If you are under the care of a physician, you should discuss any major changes in your regimen with him or her. Because this is a book and not a medical consultation, keep in mind that the information presented here may not apply in your particular case. In view of individual medical requirements, new research, and government regulations, it is the responsibility of the reader to validate health practices and treatments with a physician or health service.

Table of Contents

1

Why I Wrote This Book

I love cooking with culinary herbs – they impart such beautiful scents in the kitchen while I am preparing food and intensify the flavors of many dishes. They can also greatly enhance the enjoyment of our meals. The flavoring qualities of herbs that I enjoy include the sweetness of licorice tea, pungent curries prepared with turmeric and the spiciness of ginger, all of which delights my nose and taste buds. Many kitchen herbs can take every-day dishes like roast chicken or pasta with tomato sauce and elevate them to the most delicious ambrosia. I always keep my kitchen cupboard well stocked with a variety of delicious herbs and spices.

Herbs and spices come from plant sources and are derived from many different parts of the plant itself. Common herbs originate from the root of plants (ginger, licorice), leaves (basil, dill, tarragon, oregano), seeds (mustard, poppy, celery), and berries (black pepper, cayenne). Here is a chart that gives you some examples of the parts of the plant from which we derive many common herbs and spices.

Plant Sources of Herbs and Spices

<u>Leaves</u>

Basil

Chamomile

Dill

Oregano

Peppermint

Rosemary

Tarragon

Turmeric

<u>Roots</u>

Cinnamon

Ginger

Licorice

<u>Seeds</u>

Celery

Cumin

Mustard

Poppy

<u>Berries</u>

Black pepper

Cayenne

The Medicinal Benefits of Many Herbs and Spices

Yet, numerous culinary herbs and spices also have profound medicinal properties and can be a very beneficial addition to your therapeutic health programs. For example, many herbs such as peppermint, ginger, oregano, turmeric and cinnamon have been researched scientifically and found to have significant medicinal value. Peppermint is beneficial as an antispasmodic, chamomile as a relaxant, ginger and turmeric as anti-inflammatory agents, oregano as an antimicrobial, and cinnamon for the treatment of diabetes. Dozens of other examples of culinary herbs with medicinal properties are also discussed in this book.

Many other herbs are used strictly for their medicinal benefits. While not delicious enough to enhance the flavor of your favorite dishes and recipes, (and sometimes they can be downright unpleasant to the taste buds), they can also have dramatic beneficial effects on your health. In fact, many herbs not only help to relieve the symptoms, but also treat the causes, of many common health issues. These medicinal herbs can be kept in the pantry along with your other nutritional supplements like vitamins and minerals.

I have frequently recommended medicinal herbs in my clinical practice as part of my nutritional programs and many of my patients have found them to be effective and powerful remedies. I have also been very excited to see the explosion of medical and scientific research on the medicinal benefits of herbs.

Herbs have long been the province of traditional and folk medicine, but many Western doctors are now turning their attention to their many uses and benefits. Several universities, including UCLA and Columbia, have even hosted conferences on how to incorporate both European and Chinese herbs into standard treatment protocols. Many research studies on herbs have also been published in medical and scientific journals.

Based on my own positive clinical experience with herbs and following the exciting medical and scientific research on herbs throughout my career. I was very excited to write this book to share some of this great knowledge and information with you. My goal is to give you the best information on medicinal herbs so that you can successfully incorporate them into your own healing program.

How to Work With Herbs

Herbal seasonings and spices tend to lose their potency fairly rapidly. In fact, the more aromatic they are, the more readily this occurs. To preserve their flavoring and scent, all spices should be stored in tightly covered jars and containers, away from sunlight. Unused spices sitting on the shelf should be replaced after six months since their potency tends to fade after this period of time. Bulk herbs available in natural food stores tend to be much less expensive than pre-bottled herbs in supermarkets but often don't store as well.

Herbs and spices are also available as liquid extracts. These products capture the flavor of plants such as vanilla bean, peppermint, lemon, and almond and are sold in alcohol or water mixtures. Thus, the essence of the plant is concentrated with little nutrient value. Extracts can be very useful as flavoring agents for baked goods, frozen desserts, candies, and beverages.

Medicinal extracts often don't have the delicious flavoring that cooking herbs impart, although they can be very powerful and effective when used in healing. Like the herbs and spices themselves, extracts should be kept out of sunlight and stored in dark glass bottles to prevent rapid aging of the product. Many medicinal herbs and spices are also available in capsules as nutritional supplements available in health food stores or through the internet.

The Use of Medicinal Herbs is Not for Everyone

I do, however, want to give a caution on the use of herbs. Not everyone has the capacity to handle or tolerate medicinal herbs and should avoid their use. For example, the use of herbs in individuals with impaired detoxification capabilities can be a double-edged sword: Certain herbs have very powerful liver-cleansing and restorative effects. However, some women may not be able to process these herbs, which then overwhelm the very detoxification system that needs to be strengthened.

These women may have immediate unpleasant side effects when using medicinal herbs such as nausea, abdominal bloating, and congestion, and discomfort in the region of the liver. Such women should avoid the use of liver-cleansing herbs entirely until their detoxification capability is greatly strengthened.

If you want to try an herbal program and are unsure of your tolerance for herbs, start with one-quarter of the suggested dosages. If this is well tolerated, you can gradually increase your intake over several weeks to therapeutic levels.

2

Herbs for Healthy Digestion

Herbs and spices are time-honored digestive aids. Many of my patients use herbal teas as a healthy and satisfying alternative to acidic coffee. I also have many patients who drink coffee in the morning for a quick energy boost. However, this boost is only temporary; after an hour or two, most individuals have difficulty staying alert enough to focus on work and meet deadlines without drinking additional coffee. Ginger and peppermint teas are made from mildly stimulating herbs and can produce more subtle but sustained increases in energy. Many herbs can be used as a delicious morning beverage and have beneficial effects on both mental alertness and digestive function without causing the side effects and addiction of caffeine.

Peppermint tea also helps alleviate gas by acting as a stomach sedative and powerful antispasmodic. Chamomile tea soothes the digestive tract and also acts as a natural antispasmodic, reducing pain and discomfort. Fennel disperses gas and dispels bloating. (For this purpose, a traditional Indian curry dinner ends with a bowl of fennel.) Finally, licorice, the sweet-tasting herb used to flavor candy, has been found to be quite effective in the treatment of peptic ulcers. Research studies have shown that licorice strengthens the protective lining of the intestinal tract and helps to prevent ulcer formation.

Peppermint

Peppermint is a natural hybrid of the two mints, garden spearmint and water mint. Both peppermint and spearmint are used in herbal healing and have similar effects, but peppermint is somewhat tastier and more potent. Especially because it is a digestive, peppermint tea is often enjoyed at the end of a meal. The medicinal component of peppermint is a volatile oil. There are more than forty compounds in the oil; menthol, flavonoids, tocopherols, carotenes, and choline are just some of the substances that contribute to its therapeutic effect.

Peppermint has been used traditionally to cleanse and strengthen the entire system, including the nerves. A bath containing peppermint oil is said to be calming. Peppermint also has an antispasmodic effect on smooth muscle. Calcium in muscle cells causes the muscles to contract. Peppermint blocks this influx, which might explain why peppermint has relaxant properties. Peppermint is a suitable treatment for upset stomach and intestinal spasm. As a stomach sedative, it also helps relieve gas.

In a study appearing in *Phytomedicine*, thirty patients (twelve female and eighteen male) received the herbal drug Lomatol, containing peppermint leaves, while sixteen males and fourteen females received metoclopramide hydrochloride drops (a medication used to relieve heartburn and heal ulcers). Each patient was instructed to take twenty-five drops of the preparation in water twenty minutes before each meal, three times a day for two weeks. By the seventh day, gastrospasms were eliminated in nearly 90 percent of the patients using Lomatol, compared with only 50 percent of the patients on the hydrochloride compound.

Suggested Dosage: Peppermint is commonly taken as a tea, prepared with 1 to 2 tsp. of the dried leaves per one cup of water. Be sure to use the organic dried leaves that are available in bulk or organic leaves prepackaged in tea bags. Peppermint oil and menthol, when applied topically, can cause contact dermatitis in sensitive persons. Pregnant women are advised to use peppermint only in diluted, beverage-tea concentrations, not potent medicinal infusions. Moreover, the use of peppermint during pregnancy is discouraged for women with a history of miscarriage.

Chamomile

Chamomile is a time-honored herb, called "ground apple" by the ancient Greeks because of its pleasant apple-like scent. Chamomile was used as a stewing herb during the Middle Ages, and today it is enjoyed as a tea by both adults and children throughout Europe and Latin America. Used medicinally as a relaxant, chamomile calms nerves and promotes sleep, a benefit documented scientifically since the 1950s. The active principles of chamomile include flavonoids, glycosides, and essential oils.

As a relaxant, chamomile depresses the central nervous system, reducing anxiety while not disrupting normal performance or function. Chamomile seems an ideal herb to have on hand, given the demands and pace of modern life. Anyone who is overwhelmed by the demands of running a household while also engaging in a demanding career might benefit from a relaxing chamomile tea break. A calming drink, rather than a cup of coffee, can sometimes better restore clear thinking and the ability to work efficiently. A cup of warm chamomile tea can also temper a child's restlessness.

Chamomile also acts as an antispasmodic, helping to relax muscles that can automatically tighten when the fight-or-flight response is activated. As a tonic, chamomile can help prevent stress-related stomach cramps, poor digestion, and irritable-bowel syndrome.

Suggested Dosage: There are two types of chamomile, German (or Hungarian) and Roman (or English), both of which produce the same effects. To take as a tea, make an infusion of 2 to 3 heaping tsp. of chamomile flowers per one cup of boiling water. Let steep for ten to twenty minutes. Drink up to three cups a day. Children under the age of two may be given a weaker infusion. For a chamomile bath, tie a bunch of chamomile flowers into a cloth hung from the tub faucet, and run the bath water through it.

Ginger root

Ginger is a pungent, spicy herb native to southern Asia. For thousands of years, ginger has been an important herb used in traditional Asian medicine. It is now cultivated throughout the tropics in countries as diverse as Jamaica, India, and China. It is used as a spice in many cuisines and as a flavoring agent for beverages such as ginger ale and in many baked goods.

Ginger has thick, underground stems (tuberous rhizomes), and it is these knotted and branched rhizomes, commonly called the "root," which are used in cooking and for medicinal purposes. Records of its use in China date to the fourth century B.C. It has definite digestive benefits. As an antispasmodic, ginger is effective in relieving the nausea and vomiting associated with motion sickness and morning sickness in pregnancy. The most pharm-acologically active compounds in ginger are the various "pungent" principles, aromatic ketones known collectively as gingerols.

As for its effects on stress management, the ginger root helps stabilize blood sugar levels, preventing the mood swings that erratic highs and lows of blood glucose can trigger. Ginger also increases the efficiency of the digestive processes and thereby the availability of essential nutrients needed for proper maintenance of blood glucose.

I also have many patients who drink coffee in the morning for a quick energy boost. However, this boost is only temporary; after an hour or two, my patients report that they have difficulty staying alert enough to focus on work and meet deadlines without drinking additional cups of coffee. Ginger and peppermint teas are made from mildly stimulating herbs and can produce more subtle but sustained increases in energy

Suggested Dosage: Mix 1/2 tsp. ground ginger or 1 to 2 tsp. grated fresh ginger with 1 tsp. honey. Add one cup of boiling water to make a cup of ginger tea. You can also make a larger pot of brewed ginger tea and sip on it throughout the day. I recommend 2-3 tbsp chopped ginger added to 5 cups boiling water. Let simmer for 20 minutes.

Dry, powdered ginger root can be used in dosages of 500 to 1000 mg per day. Tripling or quadrupling this dosage may provide more rapid relief. However, dosages should not be used beyond this level.

Fennel

Fennel is a slightly sweet aromatic and flavorful herb that was widely cultivated in the Mediterranean region and often used in Italian cuisine. It is composed of a white or pale green bulb from which stalks with large feathery delicious green leaves arise, topped by flowers which produce fennel seeds.

Fennel seeds are known for their licorice flavor which many people find to be quite pleasant and delicious. Fennel's licorice flavor comes from an aromatic compound called anethole that is also found in anise and star anise. Fennel was one of the three main herbs used to create absinthe, which in the 19th century was a very popular alcoholic drink in France and other countries. In terms of its culinary uses, the bulb, leaves and seeds are used in many different culinary traditions in countries throughout the world.

Fennel has traditionally been prized for its digestive benefits. Fennel seeds have traditionally been used in India after meals, the seeds chewed to support healthy digestion and to sweeten the breath. Its most popular use is as a carminative, an herb used to prevent the formation of gas in the intestinal tract or as an antiflatulent, to help expel gas from the intestinal tract and reduce bloating. Several studies have found that fennel seed oil or fennel tea can be useful in reducing colic in infants.

It contains anethole which has been shown in animal studies to have anti-inflammatory properties, potentially reducing inflammation of the stomach and intestines. Fennel is also known to contain substances that stimulate bile, relieve pain, act as a diuretic and have antimicrobial properties.

Suggested Dosage: According to the University of Pittsburgh Medical Center, fennel may be used in the dosage of ½ teaspoon of the seeds taken two to three times a day in a tea or capsule. It can also be used as a tincture taken 1 to 2 teaspoons twice a day between meals. Fennel does produce estrogen-like effects on the body so it's used should be avoided in women with breast cancer or other estrogen stimulated health issues.

Licorice Root

The use of licorice has a long history, appearing prominently in the first great Chinese herbal The Pen Tsao Ching (Classic of Herbs), written more than 5000 years ago. Licorice today is one of the most prescribed herbs in the Chinese pharmacopoeia, second only to ginseng. Licorice has also long been used in the West for medicinal purposes. Bundles of licorice were found amid the treasures of King Tut's tomb, and licorice appears in European herbals (an herbal is a book about plants) from the Renaissance to modern times, usually prescribed and referenced as a diuretic.

The primary active component in licorice is glycyrrhizin, which has a broad range of benefits. The licorice root is fifty times sweeter than sugar. In studies, licorice has been used effectively to control hepatitis and improve liver function in people with cirrhosis.

Contemporary herbalists recommend licorice for its soothing effects on the respiratory and gastrointestinal tracts. In a study published in *The Lancet*, fifty patients with gastric ulcers were successfully treated with licorice, which was as effective as treatment with a drug such as cimetidine. Licorice also has important anti-inflammatory properties. It stimulates cell production of interferon, the body's own antiviral compound. Licorice can also be used in nutritional programs to treat bacterial and fungal infections.

Suggested Dosage: Licorice is included in the FDA's list of herbs generally regarded as safe. Overdose reports have involved highly concentrated licorice extracts used in some candies, laxatives, and tobacco products. There have been no reports of problems caused by licorice sticks or the powdered herb. However, licorice should not be used by pregnant and nursing women or by anyone with a history of diabetes, glaucoma, high blood pressure, stroke, or heart disease, as licorice can cause water retention and a rise in blood pressure.

To take licorice as a tea, gently boil ½ tsp. of the powdered herb in one cup of water for ten minutes. Drink up to two cups a day. Licorice root is also available in 300 mg capsules; take one capsule between meals two times per day. Large amounts of licorice should, however, be avoided since it can worsen high blood pressure and create low potassium levels.

Curcumin (Turmeric)

Traditional ethnic foods are often flavored with spices that have medicinal properties, which is good reason for regularly including more exotic dishes in your diet. Turmeric, an essential ingredient in curry powder, is a perennial herb of the ginger family and is extensively cultivated in India, China, Indonesia, and other tropical countries. Curcumin is the active medicinal ingredient contained in the thick rhizome of turmeric and gives turmeric its characteristic orange-yellow color. For thousands of years, curcumin has been used in both Chinese and Indian systems of medicine as an anti-inflammatory agent and for the treatment of numerous health conditions. Modern research corroborates its use as an anti-inflammatory. An article on curcumin, published in the *American Journal of Natural Medicine*, summarized several studies done in India that document curcumin's usefulness as an anti-inflammatory agent.

In one clinical trial, patients with rheumatoid arthritis were given either curcumin (1200 mg per day) or phenylbutazone (300 mg per day), an anti-inflammatory drug known to have serious side effects. The patients were then assessed for the length of time they were able to walk, persistence of morning stiffness, and degree of swelling in the joints. When the results were tabulated, the researchers found curcumin to be as beneficial as the drug therapy in reducing symptoms.

In another study, curcumin was also found to be as effective as cortisone, a potent medical anti-inflammatory. This article noted that an added benefit of curcumin is that it does not normally cause side effects, providing a safe alternative to these powerful anti-inflammatory drugs, which can cause gastric irritation and even peptic ulcers in susceptible people. Curcumin's therapeutic benefits occur through several mechanisms. Curcumin reduces inflammation by inhibiting leukotriene formation and platelet aggregation. It also promotes the breakup of blood clots and inhibits the inflammatory response to various stimuli. There is some indication that curcumin has an indirect effect on reducing inflammation through the adrenal gland or its hormones. The most likely explanation is that it increases the effectiveness of the body's own cortisone, one of the body's major anti-inflammatory hormones.

Curcumin may do this by sensitizing or priming cortisone receptor sites, thereby potentiating cortisone's action. It may also act by increasing the half-life of cortisone through reducing its breakdown by the liver. While the long-term use of prescription cortisone has been associated with serious side effects, including adrenal atrophy, osteoporosis, and diabetes mellitus, curcumin has been found to be as effective as cortisone with no toxicity.

Suggested Dosage: The recommended dosage for curcumin as an anti-inflammatory agent is 400 to 600 mg three times a day. It is often formulated with an equal amount of bromelain to enhance absorption. This combination is best taken on an empty stomach, twenty minutes before meals or between meals. Toxicity reactions have not been reported at standard dosage levels. Since curcumin has blood thinning effects, its use should be avoided in people on blood thinning drugs like Coumadin.

3

Herbs for Healthy Detoxification

Detoxification is one of our body's most crucial functions. Detoxification refers to the process of neutralizing or transforming substances that would normally be poisonous or harmful, and eliminating them from the body. Without proper detoxification, toxic substances would accumulate within the body and impair our health by interfering with the function of all our vital organ systems. Many women's health issues like PMS, fibroid tumors of the uterus, menopause symptoms, endometriosis, autoimmune disease as well as other health issues are linked to poor detoxification.

The following herbs are proven tonics for the liver and assist in healthy detoxification. They have a wide range of therapeutic benefits. Many herbs increase the flow of bile from the liver. They also stimulate increased blood flow through the liver, removing debris, old cells, and toxins. These herbs also protect the liver from a wide variety of everyday environmental toxins, such as cleaning agents and cigarette smoke, and encourage the production of enzymes that facilitate detoxification. Some of these herbs stimulate the growth of new liver cells when there is damage to the liver.

I recommend that the herbs discussed in this section be taken primarily as capsules or as teas (if palatable). I do not advise the use of tinctures and extracts for my patients with liver conditions or for those who are attempting to restore liver function if the tinctures and extracts are processed with and preserved in alcohol. Alcohol, of course, adds to the toxic load of the liver and should be avoided when using herbs for liver restoration.

Silymarin

Milk thistle plant has been used for centuries as an herbal medicine. A group of the most potent and medicinally active flavonoids found in the seed of the milk thistle plant are known collectively as silymarin. In Europe, silymarin has long been prescribed for both acute and chronic liver disease. Its effectiveness has been confirmed by more than 300 studies.

Silymarin is used to treat jaundice, cirrhosis, fatty liver, hepatitis, and congestion of the bile ducts, as well as disorders of the spleen, gallbladder, and digestive tract. In a double-blind study published in the *Scandinavian Journal of Gastroenterology*, forty-seven patients, primarily with alcohol-induced liver disease, showed significant improvement with silymarin treatment. This was evidenced by a reduction in the enzymes SGPT and SGOT, which become elevated when the liver is damaged.

Silymarin protects the liver from environmental pollutants, including smoke from tobacco, coal, oil, and incense; X-rays and the side effects of radiation therapy; and industrial toxins including carbon tetrachloride.

Animal studies demonstrate silymarin's action to be comparable to that of penicillin in counteracting poisons. There is also some documentation of silymarin's ability to protect against non-melanoma skin cancer and leukemia. Studies indicate that silymarin functions as a powerful antioxidant, scavenging free radicals that can damage liver cells. It also inhibits depletion of glutathione, one of the liver's most important antioxidant enzymes.

When liver cells are damaged by poisons, silymarin accelerates the rate of protein synthesis and regeneration of liver cells. It also prevents the reabsorption of poisons once they leave the liver and pass through the gastrointestinal tract. This reduces the toxic load on the liver and spares the cells not yet poisoned so that they can act as centers for the generation of new liver cells. With time, complete restoration of the liver is possible.

Suggested Dosage: Milk Thistle extract is considered completely safe to take in normally prescribed amounts. However, some people may experience loose stools during the first few days of taking this herb. Products containing milk thistle extract in combination with other liver restorative herbs are also available. Milk thistle extract is combined in these products with herbs such as turmeric, artichoke leaf, dandelion, or licorice. Milk thistle extract standardized to 80 percent silymarin is available in 150 to 175 mg capsules. Take one to three capsules per day.

Dandelion

Dandelion, which can grow rampant in your lawn, is a low-growing perennial plant used medicinally for over a thousand years. Arab physicians in the tenth century prescribed dandelion as a diuretic, and by the seventeenth century the English herbalist, Nicholas Culpepper incorporated dandelion as the foundation of many medicinal remedies. The early English colonists introduced dandelion to North America, where it grows in many regions of the continent.

Dandelion is often prescribed to help detoxify the liver and also to prevent gallstones. Dandelion increases the flow of bile from the liver, facilitating the detoxification process. This is supported by

German research, and German physicians routinely prescribe dandelion to prevent gallstones. Herbalists also often use dandelion, because of its diuretic properties, in the treatment of conditions involving fluid retention, such as PMS, obesity, high blood pressure, and congestive heart failure. As a diuretic, dandelion helps eliminate toxins from the body via the urine. It is also high in easily assimilated minerals, adding to its benefits.

Suggested Dosage: Dandelion is included in the FDA's list of herbs generally regarded as safe. In sensitive individuals, dandelion may cause a skin rash. It should not be used by women who are pregnant or nursing. When used as a food, dandelion leaves can be enjoyed in a salad. Mixed with other greens, they lend a tasty, slightly bitter sharpness. The leaves can also be taken as an infusion. Make a tea using ½ oz. of dried leaves per one cup of boiling water and steep ten minutes, drinking a maximum of three cups a day. Dandelion is also available in 150 mg capsules. Take one to three capsules per day.

Artichoke

The artichoke is a thistle-like plant that actually belongs to the daisy family. It is prescribed extensively in Europe to protect against toxins and to encourage the regeneration of liver cells. The principal active compound in artichokes is cynarin.

Artichoke helps prevent the accumulation of fats in the liver and arteries and is used in the treatment of atherosclerosis and arteriosclerosis. In a controlled trial published in *Drug Research,* two groups of thirty patients with hyperlipidemia (elevated blood fat levels) were treated for fifty days with cynarin (500 mg) or a placebo. Cynarin produced a significant reduction in blood cholesterol levels, lipoprotein levels, and body weight. Artichoke is also effective in preventing elevated cholesterol when toxins such as alcohol are present. As a bile stimulant, artichoke can also help prevent gallstones and liver damage from environmental toxins.

Cynarin decreases the rate of cholesterol synthesis in the liver and increases its conversion into bile acids. It also facilitates the flow of bile from the gallbladder and increases the contractive power of the bile ducts. In studies, artichoke has been shown to increase the production and volume of bile flow by as much as four times in a twelve-hour period. Artichoke also interrupts the enterohepatic circuit that would other-wise recirculate toxins between the gastrointestinal tract and the liver. Finally, artichoke stimulates the regeneration of liver cells.

Suggested Dosage: Artichoke is generally recognized as safe by the FDA. Persons who are experiencing an acute episode of pain and spasm due to inflammation of the gallbladder should not take artichoke as it may aggravate the symptoms. Artichoke is available in 160 mg capsules; take one to two capsules three times per day.

Turmeric

Turmeric is an indispensable part of the mixture of spices known as curry powder. The medicinally active compound in turmeric is curcumin, the rich orange-yellow pigment that gives turmeric its characteristic color. Turmeric has been used for thousands of years in Indian cooking and in India's traditional Ayurvedic medicine. The turmeric plant, grown from India to Indonesia, is related to ginger and has pulpy, orange, tuberous roots that grow to about two feet in length.

Turmeric is widely used in indigenous medicine in the treatment of jaundice and liver disease. Herbalists prescribe it to prevent liver damage from alcohol and other toxins. Turmeric is also known to promote circulation, dissolve blood clots, and treat irregular menstruation of all kinds.

Animal studies have shown curcumin to be an effective treatment for acute and chronic infla-mmation, and curcumin is used in the treatment of gallstones, acute and chronic inflammation of the gallbladder, and inflammation of the bile duct. In India it is applied topically to treat fresh wounds, bruises, and insect bites.

In a study in the *Journal of Nutrition*, curcumin lowered serum and liver cholesterol by one-half to one-third. Turmeric is also used as a digestive aid, facilitating the digestion of fats—hence its medicinal usefulness in curry.

Curcumin increases bile secretion and the contraction of the gallbladder, thereby facilitating detoxification and potentially lowering cholesterol. Curcumin also functions as an anti-inflammatory and anticoagulant agent. It has been shown to increase levels of glutathione-S-transferase and UDP glucuronyl transferase, 2 liver enzymes important for the promotion of phase II detoxification reactions. In addition, curcumin has been shown to have an antibacterial action and to block tumor growth.

Suggested Dosage: Turmeric is on the FDA's list of herbs generally regarded as safe. However, because turmeric has a potential anticlotting effect, anyone with a blood-clotting problem or who is currently taking anticoagulant medications should consult with their physician before taking this herb. Turmeric should not be taken by pregnant or nursing women. Turmeric is available in 400 or 500 mg capsules; take one capsule two to three times per day.

Licorice Root

The use of licorice has a long history, appearing prominently in the first great Chinese herbal The Pen

Tsao Ching (Classic of Herbs), written more than 5000 years ago. Licorice today is one of the most prescribed herbs in the Chinese pharmacopoeia, second only to ginseng. Licorice has also long been used in the West for medicinal purposes. Bundles of licorice were found amid the treasures of King Tut's tomb, and licorice appears in European herbals (an herbal is a book about plants) from the Renaissance to modern times, usually prescribed and referenced as a diuretic.

The primary active component in licorice is glycyrrhizin, which has a broad range of benefits. The licorice root is fifty times sweeter than sugar. In studies, licorice has been used effectively to control hepatitis and improve liver function in people with cirrhosis.

Contemporary herbalists recommend licorice for its soothing effects on the respiratory and gastrointestinal tracts. In a study published in *The Lancet*, fifty patients with gastric ulcers were successfully treated with licorice, which was as effective as treatment with a drug such as cimetidine. Licorice also has important anti-inflammatory properties. It stimulates cell production of interferon, the body's own antiviral compound. Licorice can also be used in nutritional programs to treat bacterial and fungal infections.

Suggested Dosage: Licorice is included in the FDA's list of herbs generally regarded as safe. Overdose reports have involved highly concentrated licorice extracts used in some candies, laxatives, and tobacco products. There have been no reports of problems caused by licorice sticks or the powdered herb.

However, licorice should not be used by pregnant and nursing women or by anyone with a history of diabetes, glaucoma, high blood pressure, stroke, or heart disease, as licorice can cause water retention and a rise in blood pressure.

To take licorice as a decoction, gently boil ½ tsp. of the powdered herb in one cup of water for ten minutes. Drink up to two cups a day. Licorice root is also available in 300 mg capsules; take one capsule between meals two times per day.

4

Herbs for Diabetes Mellitus

Diabetes Mellitus is a group of metabolic diseases in which individuals have high blood sugar. This occurs either because the body does not produce enough insulin to clear the sugar from the blood circulation or the cells of the body do not respond to the insulin that is produced by the pancreas.

Diabetes is becoming more and more prevalent in our society and, if not properly treated and controlled, can cause severe complications including nerve disorders, kidney failure, heart disease and blindness. Thus, proper treatment of diabetes is extremely important in order to maintain a high quality of life. Besides the traditional treatments of insulin and oral medication, herbs also offer benefits in diabetes control. I describe several of these herbs in this chapter.

Cinnamon

This is a sweet and delicious spice that is obtained from the brown inner bark of trees of the genus Cinnamomum. It is grown both in South East Asia and China. The use of cinnamon goes back far in antiquity. It is mentioned in the Bible and was imported to Egypt as far back as 2000 B.C. Cinnamon was also used by the ancient Greeks. It is prized during our own times for the delicious, sweet flavor that it imparts to foods and beverages. I love to bake with cinnamon, sprinkle it on toast or add it to tea. Cinnamon is one of my favorite spices.

Cinnamon has benefits for the treatment of type 2 diabetes or adult-onset diabetes which is characterized by high blood sugar levels due to insufficient insulin production by the beta cells of the pancreas insulin deficiency along with insulin resistance in which the cells of the body. The symptoms of type 2 diabetes are excessive thirst, frequent urination and increased hunger. 90% of diabetes cases are due to type 2 diabetes.

This delicious spice appears to help people with type 2 diabetes improve their ability to respond to insulin. Both test tube and animal studies have found that cinnamon stimulates insulin receptors and also inhibits the activity of an enzyme that inactivates them. This increases the cells ability to utilize glucose. Human studies are also confirming the benefit of cinnamon for diabetes.

In one study published in the journal *Diabetes*, dosages of less than ¼ of a teaspoon, ½, and 1 teaspoon per day of cinnamon were given to 60 volunteers. After 40 days all of these dosages showed benefits. These benefits included reducing the fasting blood sugar levels between 18% to 29%, total cholesterol by 12 to 26%, LDL cholesterol by 7 to 27% and triglycerides by 23% to 30%. This is significant since all of these indicators represent risk factors for heart attack as well as diabetes mellitus.

Another study tested the effect of cinnamon on 79 people who were taking oral medication to control their diabetes (rather than insulin.) They were given 3 grams of cinnamon per day or a placebo during this four month study. Again, benefits were seen with the use of cinnamon in reducing the blood sugar level versus the placebo.

A study published in the *American Journal of Clinical Nutrition* found that adding cinnamon to a high carbohydrate food slowed the rate at which the stomach emptied after eating, thereby reducing the rise in the blood sugar level.

In this study, test subjects were given either rice pudding with 6 grams (a little more than 1 teaspoon) of cinnamon added to the meal or rice pudding alone. The addition of the cinnamon was found to lower the emptying rate of the stomach by approximately 37%, thereby lowering the blood sugar level.

Suggested Dosage: ½ to 1 teaspoon of cinnamon powder per day. Sprinkle cinnamon on cereal, toast, yogurt, applesauce, juice or make a tea using cinnamon. Be cautious in using cinnamon if you are already using insulin or oral diabetic medication. Blood sugar may need to be monitored more frequently and carefully if you use cinnamon and are already on medication. Ask your doctor about using cinnamon in these circumstances.

Gymnema Sylvestre

A large, woody climbing plant, gymnema sylvestre is found in central and southern India, the tropical areas of Africa and Australia. It has been used in traditional herbal medicine for the treatment of diabetes mellitus for nearly 2000 years.

When chewing the leaves of this interesting plant, the sensation of sweetness is suppressed. In fact, it reduces the taste of sugar in the mouth for about two hours. The active ingredients creating this effect are triterpenoid saponins called gymnemic acids. (Saponins produce a soap-like foaming when shaken in water-based solutions.)

Research from in vitro studies in mouse and human beta cells, the cells that produce insulin in the pancreas, suggest that gymnema sylvestre may help to stimulate insulin secretion. Other studies found that substances in this plant decreased the uptake of sugar from the small intestine. Research done on rabbits found that gymnema sylvestre improved glucose uptake in muscle and liver as well as the storage and utilisation of sugar in the body.

A systematic review of the benefits of this plant for diabetes mellitus was published in *The Journal of Alternative and Complementary Medicine* and written by a professor from the School of Health Sciences at the University of South Australia. In reviewing the studies to date, the author found that gymnema sylvestre appears to have multiple benefits for diabetes, helping to control chronic inflammation, obesity, enzymatic defects, and pancreatic beta cell function.

Suggested Dosage: 400 mg. standardized to 25% gymnemic acids. Taken once or twice a day with meals. Gymnema sylvestre appears to be safe without significant side-effects.

5

Herbs That Improve Immune Function

Several different herbs assist in the treatment of infectious disease by improving the immune function of the body. They can be very useful as part of a complete immune boosting, anti-infection program or even when used with medication. I have found medicinal herbs to be very beneficial in a number of patients who were prone towards many types of infectious problems.

Echinacea

Echinacea root has long been used in traditional botanical medicine for its immunity-enhancing properties. In recent years, a number of studies have confirmed the beneficial effects that echinacea has on immune response, particularly against respiratory conditions like colds and flus.

Research studies have found that using echinacea increases phagocytosis (the process by which cells of the immune system engulf and destroy pathogenic organisms), activates macrophages to destroy pathogenic organisms, and stimulates both T lymphocytes and B lymphocytes.

In a review article published in the *European Journal of Herbal Medicine*, the author summarized the findings of six clinical trials using echinacea for the treatment of colds and flus as well as six trials that evaluated echinacea for its preventive benefits. The results of these trials confirmed that echinacea improves immune function when used for the treatment of respiratory infections.

Suggested Dosage: Take two capsules three times per day (125 mg capsules that have been standardized to 3.2 percent to 4.8 percent echinacosides), or take ten to thirty drops of liquid extract three times per day standardized for 1 percent echinacosides.

Oregano

Oregano is a delicious culinary herb that is commonly used in Italian cuisine in the United States. It is used in such popular foods as pizza and spaghetti and tomato sauce based dishes. It became popular in the United States during World War II when many soldiers stationed in Europe tasted dishes made with this herb while in Italy. Oregano is also used in other cuisines, including Middle Eastern, Greek, Spanish, Portuguese and Latin American countries.

Oregano's medicinal properties were recognized as far back as the Ancient Greeks. Hippocrates used oregano as a treatment for respiratory and stomach ailments. It has been shown to have antimicrobial benefits again strains of Listeria monocytogenes, a food-born pathogen.

Oil of oregano is commonly used to treat acne, which results from skin infections caused by bacteria, candida infections, parasitic infections, colds, and sore throats. It is also used to treat mild indigestion which may have some basis in animal studies and has antioxidant benefits which have been confirmed in several research studies.

Suggested Dosage: Take 1 to 3 drops of the oil one to three times a day under the tongue

Garlic

Garlic is a delicious and pungent culinary herb, used throughout the world. It is renowned for its strong aroma and flavor. Besides being an important component of American and European cooking, garlic is also commonly used in the cuisines of the Middle East, Asia, northern Africa, and parts of South and Central America. Its use goes back to ancient Egypt during the times of the building of the pyramids and the ancient Greeks.

In modern times, entire festivals, like the Gilroy Garlic Festival in California, the Minnesota Garlic Festival and Pocono Garlic Festival in Pennsylvania are held each year. These, and many other festivals in different parts of the country, are dedicated to garlic used in every possible type of dish including garlic ice cream!

Garlic bulbs are primarily used in recipes and become more mellow and sweeter with cooking. Some recipes, like dips such as hummus or baba ganoush, often use raw garlic to give a sweet and tangy flavor to the dishes. Olive oil, and other oils, can be infused with garlic and used in cooking.

Garlic cloves are also used raw, dried or cooked for its medicinal benefits. Garlic contains an organic compound, called allicin, which gives garlic its aroma and flavor and is also a very powerful antioxidant.

Research published in the chemistry journal *Angewandte Chemie* found that allicin is a very powerful and rapid acting antioxidant that destroys dangerous free radicals. This reaction occurs once allicin decomposes and produces an acid that powerfully reacts with free radicals. Although onions, leeks and shallots are in the same plant family as garlic and contain a compound similar to allicin, they do not have the same medicinal properties.

Garlic has a long history of use as an antimicrobial agent. In World War I and World War II, garlic was used as an antiseptic and antimicrobial agent to help prevent gangrene. A mouthwash containing fresh garlic was developed that showed antimicrobial activity. However, most of the study participants did not like the mouthwash because of it had an unpleasant taste and caused bad smelling breath.

In in vitro studies, garlic has been found to have antimicrobial properties. Studies have shown garlic to have antibacterial, antiviral and antifungal activity. It is often used to treat candida infections and thrush, a fungal infection of the throat. People often use garlic to prevent and treat the common cold and sinus infections, mostly based on traditional and clinical findings rather than research studies. It has also been used in China to treat cryptosporidium, a protozoa which causes gastrointestinal illnesses including symptoms of diarrhea, especially in patients infected with AIDS. People with AIDS can develop a chronic, persistent form of this disease which can be difficult to treat.

When applied topically in a cream, garlic has antifungal properties and can kill fungus including possibly even healing athlete's foot. It has also been combined with mullein in oil products. It has been found to reduce the pain, but not the actual infection, of otitis media or middle ear infections. However, the topical use of garlic may cause burning or blistering of the skin in some sensitive individuals so it should be used carefully.

Suggested Dosage: When using raw garlic, 4 grams of fresh garlic per day, which is approximately 1 clove can be effective. Garlic capsules are also available, including deodorized garlic, which is more readily tolerated by many people. **Suggested Dosage** of garlic is 900 mg per day of a garlic powder standardized to contain 1.3% allicin. Garlic may also be found in cream or oil products for topical use.

The most common side effect of garlic use is body odor, bad breath and a burning sensation in the mouth. Some people report having heartburn or diarrhea with the use of raw garlic and find that they cannot tolerate it. Garlic use should also be avoided by people on anticoagulant drugs like Coumadin because of its blood thinning properties.

It is possibly safe for pregnant and nursing mothers except just before and immediately after delivery, although this has not been definitely proven. If you have any questions or concerns, I recommend that you ask your doctor about the advisability of using garlic for your particular case.

Ginseng

Ginseng root has been used as a tonic to improve resistance to infectious disease in traditional Asian medicine for several thousand years. Research studies have confirmed that ginseng root improves immune function by stimulating the activity of natural killer cells and increasing the production of lymphocytes.

An article published in *Drugs Under Experimental and Clinical Research* discussed the results of a study in which the ability of ginseng to improve immune response to the influenza vaccine was evaluated versus a placebo. Two hundred twenty-seven adult volunteers were given either 100 mg of a standardized extract of ginseng root or a placebo daily over a twelve-week period. All of the volunteers were given an influenza vaccine at week four.

The volunteers taking the ginseng root showed a significantly greater immune response to the influenza vaccine than did the placebo group. In addition, the individuals in the treatment group experienced fewer cases of influenza and fewer colds than those in the placebo group.

Suggested Dosage: For maximum benefit, take a high-quality preparation. This means using an extract of the main root of a plant that is four to six years old, standardized for ginsenoside content and ratio. Twice a day, take a 100 mg capsule. If this is too stimulating, especially before bedtime, take the second dose midafternoon, or take only the morning dose.

6

Anti-Inflammatory Herbs

Inflammation is a major factor in many common illnesses including autoimmune diseases like rheumatoid arthritis, lupus, endometriosis, heart disease, allergies and even cancer. Autoimmune diseases are found much more commonly in women than men and can cause painful and devastating symptoms. The following herbs can be very beneficial in helping to control and reverse inflammation.

Turmeric

Turmeric has been used for thousands of years in Indian cooking and in India's traditional Ayurvedic medicine. The turmeric plant, grown from India to Indonesia, is related to ginger and has pulpy, orange, tuberous roots that grow to about two feet in length. It is an indispensable part of the mixture of spices known as curry powder. The medicinally active compound in turmeric is curcumin, the rich orange-yellow pigment that gives turmeric its characteristic orange-yellow color.

For thousands of years, curcumin has been used in both Chinese and Indian systems of medicine as an anti-inflammatory agent and for the treatment of numerous health conditions. Modern research corroborates its use as an anti-inflammatory.

A review article on curcumin, published in the *American Journal of Natural Medicine*, summarized several studies done in India that document curcumin's usefulness as an anti-inflammatory agent. In one clinical trial, patients with rheumatoid arthritis were given either curcumin (1200 mg per day) or phenylbutazone (300 mg per day), an anti-inflammatory drug known to have serious side effects. The patients were then assessed for the length of time they were able to walk, persistence of morning stiffness, and degree of swelling in the joints. When the results were tabulated, the researchers found curcumin to be as beneficial as the drug therapy in reducing symptoms.

In another study, curcumin was also found to be as effective as cortisone, a potent medical anti-inflammatory. This article noted that an added benefit of curcumin is that it does not normally cause side effects, providing a safe alternative to these powerful anti-inflammatory drugs, which can cause gastric irritation and even peptic ulcers in susceptible people.

Curcumin's therapeutic benefits occur through several mechanisms. Curcumin reduces inflammation by inhibiting leukotriene formation and platelet aggregation. It also promotes the break-up of blood clots and inhibits the inflammatory response to various stimuli. There is some indication that curcumin has an indirect effect on reducing inflammation through the adrenal gland or its hormones.

The most likely explanation is that it increases the effectiveness of the body's own cortisone, which is one of the body's major anti-inflammatory hormones. Curcumin may do this by sensitizing or priming cortisone receptor sites, thereby potentiating cortisone's action. It may also act by increasing the half-life of cortisone through reducing its breakdown by the liver. While the long-term use of prescription cortisone has been associated with serious side effects, including adrenal atrophy, osteoporosis, and diabetes mellitus, curcumin has been found to be as effective as cortisone with no toxicity.

Suggested Dosage: The recommended dosage for curcumin as an anti-inflammatory agent is 400 to 600 mg three times a day. It is often formulated with an equal amount of bromelain to enhance absorption. This combination is best taken on an empty stomach, twenty minutes before meals or between meals. Toxicity reactions have not been reported at standard dosage levels.

Since curcumin has blood thinning effects, its use should be avoided in people on blood thinning drugs like Coumadin. It should not be used by pregnant or nursing women.

Ginger

Ginger is a pungent, spicy herb native to southern Asia. For thousands of years, ginger has been an important herb used in traditional Asian medicine. It is now cultivated throughout the tropics in countries as diverse as Jamaica, India, and China. It is used as a spice in many cuisines and as a flavoring agent for beverages such as ginger ale and in many baked goods.

Ginger is a powerful anti-inflammatory agent. This herb works through modulating or balancing the prost-aglandin pathway. Chemicals in ginger have been found to inhibit inflammatory chemicals like thromboxanes and leukotrienes, which have been linked to conditions like asthma and coronary-artery spasm. On the other hand, these chemicals do not interfere with the production of beneficial anti-inflammatory prostaglandins. As a result, ginger has been found to reduce inflammation, pain, and fever in a variety of conditions. As such, its effects are similar to medications like aspirin, without the toxic side effects.

Suggested Dosage: Dry, powdered ginger root can be used in dosages of 500 to 1000 mg per day. Tripling or quadrupling this dosage may provide more rapid relief. However, dosages should not be used beyond this level.

Licorice Root

The use of licorice has a long history, appearing prominently in the first great Chinese herbal The Pen Tsao Ching (Classic of Herbs), written more than 5000 years ago. Licorice today is one of the most prescribed herbs in the Chinese pharmacopoeia, second only to ginseng. Licorice has also long been used in the West for medicinal purposes. Bundles of licorice sticks were found amid the treasures of King Tut's tomb, and licorice appears in European herbals (an herbal is a book about plants) from the Renaissance to modern times, usually prescribed and referenced as a diuretic.

The primary active component in licorice is glycyrrhizin, which has a broad range of benefits. The licorice root is fifty times sweeter than sugar. In studies, licorice has been used effectively to control hepatitis and improve liver function in people with cirrhosis.

Contemporary herbalists recommend licorice for its soothing effects on the respiratory and gastro-intestinal tracts. In a study published in *The Lancet*, fifty patients with gastric ulcers were successfully treated with licorice, which was as effective as treatment with a drug such as cimetidine. Licorice also has important anti-inflammatory properties. It stimulates cell production of interferon, the body's own antiviral compound. Licorice can also be used in nutritional programs to treat bacterial and fungal infections.

Suggested Dosage: Licorice is included in the FDA's list of herbs generally regarded as safe. Overdose reports have involved highly concentrated licorice extracts used in some candies, laxatives, and tobacco products. There have been no reports of problems caused by licorice sticks or the powdered herb. However, licorice should not be used by pregnant and nursing women or by anyone with a history of diabetes, glaucoma, high blood pressure, stroke, or heart disease, as licorice can cause water retention and a rise in blood pressure.

To take licorice as a tea, gently boil ½ tsp. of the powdered herb in one cup of water for ten minutes. Drink up to two cups a day. Licorice root is also available in 300 mg capsules; take one capsule between meals two times per day.

7

Herbs for Healthy Hearts and Circulation

The incidence of heart disease begins to increase dramatically once women reach menopause, although it can be seen even in younger women. There are a number of herbs that have powerful circulatory benefits, promoting healthy blood flow to the organs and tissues throughout the body. In addition, they can improve blood flow and oxygenation to the heart, thereby improving cardiovascular function. The anti-inflammatory qualities of certain herbs also benefit heart function and reduce coronary artery spasm. Herbs also acts as blood thinning agents, lessening the risk of clots, as well as reduce elevated blood lipids, a risk factor for heart attacks.

Garlic

Garlic is a delicious and pungent culinary herb, used throughout the world. It is renowned for its strong aroma and flavor. Besides being an important component of American and European cooking, garlic is also commonly used in the cuisines of the Middle East, Asia, northern Africa, and parts of South and Central America. Its use goes back to ancient Egypt during the times of the building of the pyramids and the ancient Greeks.

In modern times, entire festivals, like the Gilroy Garlic Festival in California, the Minnesota Garlic Festival and Pocono Garlic Festival in Pennsylvania are held each year. These, and many other festivals in different parts of the country, are dedicated to garlic used in every possible type of dish including garlic ice cream!

Garlic bulbs are primarily used in recipes and become more mellow and sweeter with cooking. Some recipes, like dips such as hummus or baba ganoush, often use raw garlic to give a sweet and tangy flavor to the dishes. Olive oil, and other oils, can be infused with garlic and used in cooking.

Garlic cloves are also used raw, dried or cooked for its medicinal benefits. Garlic contains an organic compound, called allicin, which gives garlic its aroma and flavor and is also a very powerful antioxidant.

Research published in the chemistry journal *Angewandte Chemie* found that allicin is a very powerful and rapid acting antioxidant that destroys dangerous free radicals. This reaction occurs once allicin decomposes and produces an acid that powerfully reacts with free radicals.

Although onions, leeks and shallots are in the same plant family as garlic and contain a compound similar to allicin, they do not have the same medicinal properties.

Garlic may have some benefits for individuals who are at risk for heart attacks or strokes. In one double blind, placebo controlled study of patients who were on medical treatment but had uncontrolled hypertension, garlic extract was found to lower systolic blood pressure. Other studies have found blood pressure reductions varying from five to ten percent with the use of garlic supplements.

Animal studies have shown the benefits of garlic in reducing the risk of cardiovascular disease. Garlic may slow down the development of atherosclerosis or hardening of the arteries. Both animal and human studies suggest that this may be true. Included is a study that found that garlic supplementation reduced aortic plaque deposits in cholesterol-fed rabbits. Another animal study showed that garlic reduced accumulation of cholesterol on blood vessel walls.

In a human study, a garlic extract inhibited vascular calcification in patients with elevated blood cholesterol. In a double blind, placebo controlled human study; standardized garlic powder was found to slow the development of atherosclerosis when measured by ultrasound testing. Finally, an observational study found that patients who took garlic had more flexibility in the aorta, the main artery that exits from the heart. This would be an indication of less atherosclerosis forming within the aorta.

All of these studies are quite positive, if not conclusive, in terms of garlic having a beneficial influence on cardiovascular function. Yet despite the long held belief that garlic reduces high cholesterol levels, study results have been mixed in terms of garlic normalizing blood cholesterol levels. Garlic does appear to be an anticoagulant, in other words to act as a blood thinner. This may help to prevent heart attacks and strokes.

Suggested Dosage: For the treatment of cardiovascular disease, the National Institute of Health recommends 4 grams of fresh garlic per day, which is approximately 1 clove. Garlic capsules are also available, including deodorized garlic that is more readily tolerated by many people. You can also use 900 mg per day of a garlic powder standardized to contain 1.3% allicin.

The most common side effect of garlic use is body odor, bad breath and a burning sensation in the mouth. Some people report having heartburn or diarrhea with the use of raw garlic and find that they cannot tolerate it. Garlic use should also be avoided by people on anticoagulant drugs like Coumadin because of its blood thinning properties.

It is possibly safe for pregnant and nursing mothers except just before and immediately after delivery, although this has not been definitely proven. If you have any questions about the use of garlic, I recommend that you ask your doctor about the advisability of using garlic for your particular case.

Ginger

Ginger is a pungent, spicy herb native to southern Asia. For thousands of years, ginger has been an important herb used in traditional Asian medicine. It is now cultivated throughout the tropics in countries as diverse as Jamaica, India, and China. It is used as a spice in many cuisines and as a flavoring agent for beverages such as ginger ale and in many baked goods.

Ginger is a powerful anti-inflammatory agent. It works through modulating or balancing the prostaglandin pathway. Chemicals in ginger have been found to inhibit inflammatory chemicals like thromboxanes and leukotrienes, which have been linked to conditions like asthma and coronary-artery spasm. On the other hand, these chemicals do not interfere with the production of beneficial anti-inflammatory prostaglandins. As a result, ginger has been found to reduce inflammation, pain, and fever in a variety of conditions. As such, its effects are similar to medications like aspirin, without the toxic side effects.

Ginger also acts as a vasodilator, promoting healthier blood circulation throughout the body. This beneficial property means that more oxygenation and nutrient flow reaches the heart and other essential organs of the body.

Suggested Dosage: Dry, powdered ginger root can be used in dosages of 500 to 1000 mg per day. Tripling or quadrupling this dosage may provide more rapid relief. However, dosages should not be used beyond this level.

Turmeric

Turmeric has been used for thousands of years in Indian cooking and in India's traditional Ayurvedic medicine. The turmeric plant, grown from India to Indonesia, is related to ginger and has pulpy, orange, tuberous roots that grow to about two feet in length. It is an indispensable part of the mixture of spices known as curry powder. The medicinally active compound in turmeric is curcumin, the rich orange-yellow pigment that gives turmeric its characteristic orange-yellow color.

For thousands of years, curcumin has been used in both Chinese and Indian systems of medicine as an anti-inflammatory agent and for the treatment of numerous health conditions. Modern research corroborates its use as an anti-inflammatory.

A review article on curcumin, published in the *American Journal of Natural Medicine,* summarized several studies done in India that document curcumin's usefulness as an anti-inflammatory agent.

In one study, curcumin was also found to be as effective as cortisone, a potent medical anti-inflammatory. This article noted that an added benefit of curcumin is that it does not normally cause side effects, providing a safe alternative to these powerful anti-inflammatory drugs, which can cause gastric irritation and even peptic ulcers in susceptible people.

As an antioxidant, curcumin reduces free radical damage in tissues, including the blood vessels. Its potent anti-inflammatory benefits reduce destructive reactions within the heart as well as many other tissues. A study reported in the *Indian Journal of Physiology and Pharmacology* also found curcumin to be useful in reducing the levels of total cholesterol and elevating the levels of healthy HDL cholesterol.

Curcumin's therapeutic benefits occur through several mechanisms. Curcumin reduces inflammation by inhibiting leukotriene formation and platelet aggregation. It also promotes the breakup of blood clots and inhibits the inflammatory response to various stimuli. There is some indication that curcumin has an indirect effect on reducing inflammation through the adrenal gland or its hormones.

The most likely explanation is that it increases the effectiveness of the body's own cortisone, one of the body's major anti-inflammatory hormones. Curcumin may do this by sensitizing or priming cortisone receptor sites, thereby potentiating cortisone's action. It may also act by increasing the half-life of cortisone through reducing its breakdown by the liver. While the long-term use of prescription cortisone has been associated with serious side effects, including adrenal atrophy, osteoporosis, and diabetes mellitus, curcumin has been found to be as effective as cortisone with no toxicity.

Suggested Dosage: The recommended dosage for curcumin as an anti-inflammatory agent is 400 to 600 mg three times a day. It is often formulated with an equal amount of bromelain to enhance absorption. This combination is best taken on an empty stomach, twenty minutes before meals or between meals. Toxicity reactions have not been reported at standard dosage levels.

Since curcumin is a blood thinning agent, its use should probably be avoided in people on blood thinning agents like Coumadin.

Ginkgo Biloba

The ginkgo biloba tree species originated about 250 million years ago, and a single tree can live as long as 1000 years. This handsome tree is often planted in urban settings, as it resists disease, insects, and pollution. Modern science is finding that this ancient plant can also help slow the aging of the brain, alleviate depression, and, perhaps most importantly, improve circulation and oxygenation throughout the body.

Ginkgo leaf extracts are used by individuals throughout the world for their circulatory and oxygenation benefits. The chemicals found in ginkgo have powerful vasodilating effects: They act by stimulating the release of prostacyclin (a prosta-glandin hormone) and a vascular relaxing substance. These chemicals also improve the tone of blood vessels and reduce the stickiness of red blood cells, so that they flow more smoothly through the blood vessels as they carry oxygen throughout the body.

Numerous research studies confirm the benefits of ginkgo extracts on all parts of the circulatory system, improving blood flow and oxygenation to the brain, heart, and other vital organs and the extremities. It is useful for many conditions including coronary-artery disease, cerebral vascular insufficiency, peripheral vascular disease, Alzheimer's disease, diseases of the eye due to diabetes mellitus or poor circulation, edema due to PMS, Reynaud's disease (vaso-constriction of the extremities), impotence due to diminished blood flow, cyclic and even clinical depression (gingko acts as a potent mood elevator).

Many important performance traits are enhanced by the improvement in the oxygenation of the body that occurs when using ginkgo. These include improvements in physical energy, mental clarity, cognitive function, mood, and ability to socialize. Side effects are rare; however, women should be aware that the flavonoid quercetin, which is found in ginkgo, may lower estrogen production within the body.

Suggested Dosage: Only standardized extracts should be used (standardized to 24 percent flavonoid glycosides and 6 percent terpene lactones). Dosages may vary between 40 to 60 mg, two to three times a day.

8

Herbs for Adrenal Support

Many women suffer from adrenal exhaustion which impairs their ability to work effectively and manage their busy lives. Adaptogenic herbs support the adrenals (as well as the ovaries and other endocrine glands), thereby preventing the long-term adrenal burnout and exhaustion that occurs with chronic stress.

An adaptogen is a substance that is able to safely increase resistance to a wide range of adverse physical, chemical, and biochemical factors, and promotes normalization between extremes. These herbs also contain a wide variety of chemicals that help the body recover more quickly from hard physical labor, athletic exertion, and even convalescence from surgery.

Rhodiola Rosea

Rhodiola rosea is a popular plant indigenous to Eastern Europe and Asia. The ancient Greeks used the herb medicinally as far back as 100 A.D. Named for the rose-like odor of the rootstock when newly cut, Rhodiola rosea has been used for centuries in China to prolong life and enhance wisdom. Siberian healers believe that people who drink Rhodiola tea on a regular basis will live to be more than 100 years old. And in the former Soviet Union, Rhodiola has been used to diminish fatigue and increase your body's resistance to stress.

Rhodiola works to support all hormone production by easing stress and fatigue—both destroy healthy hormone production. According to the journal *Phytomedicine*, Rhodiola is particularly effective in fighting stress-induced fatigue which depletes the adrenal glands significantly.

In one study, researchers tested 40 male medical students during exam time to determine if the herb positively affected physical fitness, as well as mental well-being and capacity. The students were divided into two groups and given either 50 mg of Rhodiola rosea extract or a placebo twice a day for 20 days. Researchers found that those students who took the extract had a significant decrease in mental fatigue and increase of psychomotor function, with a 50 percent improvement in neuromotor function. Plus, scores from exams taken immediately after the study showed that the extract group had an average grade of 3.47, as compared to 3.20 for the placebo group.

Suggested Dosage: To ease fatigue, stress, or anxiety—all of which can play havoc with your adrenal hormone production—and boost your energy and stamina (which the adrenal glands support), I recommend taking 50-100 mg of Rhodiola rosea three times a day, standardized to 3 percent rosavins and 0.8 percent salidrosides. While the herb is generally considered safe, some reports have indicated that it may counteract the effects of antiarrhythmic medications. Therefore, if you are currently taking this type of medication, I suggest you discuss the use of Rhodiola rosea with your physician.

Panax Ginseng

Panax ginseng is an ivy-like ground cover originating in the wild, damp woodlands of northern China and Korea. Its use in Chinese herbal medicine dates back more than 4000 years. In colonial North America, ginseng was a major export product. The wild form is now rare, but panax ginseng is a widely cultivated plant.

Ginseng has a legendary status among herbs. While extravagant claims have been made about its many uses, scientific research has yielded inconsistent results in verifying its therapeutic properties. However, enough good research does exist to demonstrate ginseng's activity, especially when high-quality extracts, standardized for active components, are used.

Ginseng has a balancing, tonic effect on the systems and organs of the body involved in the stress response. It contains at least thirteen different saponins, a class of chemicals found in many plants, especially legumes, which take their name from their ability to form a soap-like froth when shaken with water. These compounds (triterpene glycosides) are the most pharmaceutically active constituents of ginseng. Saponins benefit cardiovascular function, immunity, hormone production, and the central nervous system.

During times of stress, ginseng acts as a general stimulant, delaying the alarm phase in Selye's classic model of stress. The saponins in the ginseng act on the hypothalamus and pituitary glands, increasing the release of adrenocorticotrophin, or ACTH (a hormone produced by the pituitary that promotes the manufacture and secretion of adrenal hormones). As a result, ginseng increases the release of adrenal cortisone and other adrenal hormones, and prevents their depletion from stress. Other substances associated with the pituitary are also released, such as endorphins. Ginseng is used to prevent adrenal atrophy, which can be a side effect of cortisone drug treatment.

In a double-blind study published in *Drugs Under Experimental and Clinical Research*, two groups of volunteers suffering from fatigue due to physical or mental stress were given nutritional supplementation over a twelve-week period. One hundred sixty-three volunteers were given a multivitamin and multi-mineral complex, and 338 volunteers received the same product plus a standardized Chinese ginseng extract. Once a month, the volunteers were asked to fill out a questionnaire during a scheduled visit with a physician. This questionnaire contained eleven questions that asked them to describe their current level of perceived physical energy, stamina, sense of well-being, libido, and quality of sleep.

While both groups experienced similar improvement in their quality of life by the second visit, the group using the ginseng extract almost doubled their improvement, based on their responses, by the third and fourth visits. Thus, ginseng, when added to a multivitamin and multi mineral complex, appears to improve many factors of well-being in individuals experiencing significant physical and emotional stress.

Many of my patients have used ginseng and have found it to have energizing effects, especially Korean red ginseng, which is considered to be hotter (more "yang") and stronger than other forms of ginseng, including Chinese and American, which are more cooling (more "yin") and calming in their effects.

While Korean ginseng is well suited to men, women may find the effects of this form of ginseng too extreme for the female body. Women can experience extremely heightened levels of libido with the use of Korean ginseng, as well as tremendous surges of energy. However, it can also disrupt the menstrual cycle, causing a decrease in normal menstrual flow and dryness of the skin and mucous membranes. As a result, women tend to do better with Chinese or American ginseng.

There is evidence in animal and human studies that ginseng increases stamina and endurance. Studies show that ginseng prevents fatigue, lengthening the time it takes to reach exhaustion. Ginseng also enhances mental capacity, as demonstrated in both animal studies and clinical trials in humans. Improvements in logical deduction, reaction time, mental arithmetic, alertness, and accuracy have been observed. ACTH (the hormone that stimulates the adrenal cortex) and adrenal hormones, which ginseng stimulates, are known to bind to brain tissue, increasing mental activity during stress.

Suggested Dosage: For maximum benefit, take a high-quality preparation, an extract of the main root of a plant that is six to eight years old, standardized for ginsenoside content and ratio. Companies that make ginseng products may mention the age of the plants used in their products as a testimony to their products' quality. Take a 100 mg capsule twice a day. If this is too stimulating, especially before bedtime, take the second dose midafternoon, or take only the morning dose.

Siberian Ginseng

Siberian ginseng (Eleutherococcus senticosus) is part of the same family as panax ginseng, but the exact composition differs considerably. The most pharm-acologically active constituents in Siberian ginseng are eleutherosides, some of which are similar in structure to the saponins contained in Asian ginseng.

Siberian ginseng has been used in Asia for nearly 2000 years to combat fatigue and increase endurance. The medicinal properties of this plant have been studied in Russia, with a number of clinical and experimental studies demonstrating that eleuth-erosides are adaptogenic, increasing resistance to stress and fatigue.

According to a review of clinical trials of more than 2100 healthy human subjects, ranging in age from nineteen to seventy-two, published in *Economic Medicinal Plant Research*, Siberian ginseng reduces activation of the adrenal cortex in response to stress, an action useful in the alarm stage of the fight-or-flight response. It also helps lower blood pressure.

In this same study, data indicated that the eleuth-erosides increased the subjects' ability to withstand adverse physical conditions including heat, noise, motion, an increase in workload, and exercise. There was also improved quality of work under stressful work conditions and improved athletic performance. Siberian ginseng can be of benefit to athletes and also to a person working hard to meet a deadline. Ginseng may help a person push beyond their normal capacity when the only way to finish a job is to pull an all-nighter. Herbalists have also long prescribed Siberian ginseng for chronic-fatigue syndrome.

One way in which ginseng may increase energy reserves is through its ability to facilitate the conversion of fat into energy, in both intense and moderate physical activity, sparing carbohydrates and postponing the point at which a runner, for instance, may "hit the wall." This occurs when stored glucose is depleted and can no longer serve as a source of energy.

Siberian ginseng is also used to treat a variety of psychological disturbances, including insomnia, hypochondriasis, and various neuroses. The reason ginseng is effective may be its ability to balance stress hormones and neurotransmitters such as epine-phrine, serotonin, and dopamine.

Suggested Dosage: Siberian ginseng has virtually no toxicity, although individuals with fever, hypertonic crisis, or myocardial infarction are advised not to use it. A standard dosage of the fluid extract (33 percent ethanol) ranges from 2.0 to 4.0 ml, one to three times a day, for periods of up to sixty consecutive days. An equivalent dosage of dry powdered extract concentrated at a ratio of 20:1 is 100 to 200 mg. Take in multiple-dose regimens with two to three weeks between courses.

I have had a number of patients over the years who have bought inexpensive ginseng, either as a root or in capsule form, expecting miraculous results, given ginseng's venerable reputation. Unfortunately, these cheaper grades of ginseng rarely, if ever, deliver the punch that individuals expect—that is, the chemical equivalent of an auxiliary set of adrenal glands or reproductive glands.

I have, however, seen some remarkable results with high-grade ginseng purchased from reputable Chinese pharmacists that sell top-of-the-line herbs or American companies selling herbs of equivalent quality. Given that the potency of the therapeutic chemicals takes many years to develop within the ginseng root, it is no surprise that, with ginseng, you get what you pay for. Individuals with a serious interest in using ginseng for its adaptogenic properties should search out the reputable dealers.

Licorice Root

Licorice has been enjoyed over the centuries as a candy, but it is also an herb with medicinal properties, featured in the great recorded herbals for 4000 years. Respected by the ancient Egyptians, licorice was among the treasured items archaeologists discovered (in great quantities) when they opened King Tut's tomb. Sometime around the year 1600, John Josselyn of Boston listed licorice as one of the "precious herbs" brought from England to colonial America.

Licorice is used to treat respiratory conditions, urinary and kidney problems, fatty liver, hepatitis, the inflammation of arthritis, and ulcers. The herb also exhibits hormone-like activity. Licorice root increases the half-life of cortisol (the adrenal stress hormone), inhibiting the breakdown of adrenal hormones by the liver. As a result, licorice is useful in reversing low cortisol conditions and helping the adrenal glands rest and restore function.

Licorice also contains potent estrogen like chemicals. Since estrogen has profound mood-elevating effects, licorice has antidepressant properties. For a person under a variety of stresses, licorice may be the needed antidote because of its energizing and antidepressant actions.

Suggested Dosage: A standard dosage is 1 to 2 g of powdered root administered at three separate times per day. Licorice has activity similar to aldosterone, the adrenal hormone responsible for regulating water and electrolytes within the body. As a result, taking large doses of licorice (10 to 14 g of the crude herb) can lead to high blood pressure, water retention, and sodium and potassium imbalances. Licorice should not be taken by children under age two. Caution should be used with older children, pregnant and nursing women, and people over sixty-five. Start with low dosages and increase the strength only if necessary.

Gotu Kola

Gotu kola (Centella asiatica), also called centella, has been used since prehistoric times in India. It has been used both internally and externally, based on its ability to heal wounds and treat skin conditions such as eczema, varicose ulcers, and leprosy. In the 1880s, gotu kola was incorporated into the French pharmacopoeia. (American consumers sometimes confuse gotu kola and its rejuvenating activity with kola nuts, which are stimulating because they contain caffeine.) Gotu kola has an action similar to Siberian ginseng, acting as a potent anti-fatigue nutrient. People who are experiencing excessive levels of anxiety may find the energy-supporting qualities of gotu kola quite helpful.

Gotu kola was used in China to delay senility. Modern studies are beginning to confirm its effectiveness in improving mental function. It has been used to increase the mental abilities of disabled children. The primary active components of gotu kola are triterpene compounds. These are asiatic acid, madecassic acid, asiaticoside, and madecassoside. These triterpenes liberate the neurotransmitter acetylcholine, which is important for cognitive function. It is assumed that because of this, mental capacity often improves. Gotu kola also has a tranquilizing effect and counteracts stress.

Suggested Dosage: If using a standardized extract, take 60 to 120 mg per day. If taking the crude dried plant leaves, take 2 to 4 g per day.

Turmeric

Traditional ethnic foods are often flavored with spices that have medicinal properties, which is good reason for regularly including more exotic dishes in your diet. Turmeric, an essential ingredient in curry powder, is a perennial herb of the ginger family and is extensively cultivated in India, China, Indonesia, and other tropical countries. Curcumin is the active medicinal ingredient contained in the thick rhizome of turmeric and gives turmeric its characteristic orange-yellow color.

For thousands of years, curcumin has been used in both Chinese and Indian systems of medicine as an anti-inflammatory agent and for the treatment of numerous health conditions. Modern research corroborates its use as an anti-inflammatory.

A review article on curcumin, published in the *American Journal of Natural Medicine*, summarized several studies done in India that document curcumin's usefulness as an anti-inflammatory agent. In one clinical trial, patients with rheumatoid arthritis were given either curcumin (1200 mg per day) or phenylbutazone (300 mg per day), an anti-inflammatory drug known to have serious side effects. The patients were then assessed for the length of time they were able to walk, persistence of morning stiffness, and degree of swelling in the joints.

When the results were tabulated, the researchers found curcumin to be as beneficial as the drug therapy in reducing symptoms. In another study, curcumin was also found to be as effective as cortisone, a potent medical anti-inflammatory. This article noted that an added benefit of curcumin is that it does not normally cause side effects, providing a safe alternative to these powerful anti-inflammatory drugs, which can cause gastric irritation and even peptic ulcers in susceptible people.

Curcumin's therapeutic benefits occur through several mechanisms. Curcumin reduces inflammation by inhibiting leukotriene formation and platelet aggregation. It also promotes the breakup of blood clots and inhibits the inflammatory response to various stimuli.

There is some indication that curcumin has an indirect effect on reducing inflammation through the adrenal gland or its hormones. The most likely explanation is that it increases the effectiveness of the body's own cortisone, one of the body's major anti-inflammatory hormones. Curcumin may do this by sensitizing or priming cortisone receptor sites, thereby potentiating cortisone's action. It may also act by increasing the half-life of cortisone through reducing its breakdown by the liver. While the long-term use of prescription cortisone has been associated with serious side effects, including adrenal atrophy, osteoporosis, and diabetes mellitus, curcumin has been found to be as effective as cortisone with no toxicity.

Suggested Dosage: The recommended dosage for curcumin as an anti-inflammatory agent is 400 to 600 mg three times a day. It is often formulated with an equal amount of bromelain to enhance absorption. This combination is best taken on an empty stomach, twenty minutes before meals or between meals. Toxicity reactions have not been reported at standard dosage levels.

Since curcumin has blood thinning effects, its use should be avoided in people on blood thinning drugs like Coumadin.

9

Herbs for Brain Support

One of the most crucial and important organs for maintaining health and wellness in our entire body is the brain. The brain regulates almost every important physiological function within the body including intelligence, memory, speech, creativity, emotions, spirituality, our organ systems and even our female hormones.

Imbalances in brain function are commonly seen in a wide variety of health issues, including menopause, PMS, anxiety, depression, Parkinson's disease infectious diseases, chronic fatigue and many other conditions. Providing nutritional support for the brain is thus very important to maintain its health and prevent premature aging. Herbs can play an important role in achieving this goal.

Ginkgo Biloba

The ginkgo biloba tree species originated about 250 million years ago, and a single tree can live as long as 1000 years. This handsome tree is often planted in urban settings, as it resists disease, insects, and pollution. Modern science is finding that this ancient plant can also help slow the aging of the brain, alleviate depression, and, perhaps most importantly, improve circulation and oxygenation throughout the body. In fact, ginkgo leaf extracts are used by individuals throughout the world for their circulatory and oxygenation benefits.

The chemicals found in ginkgo have powerful vasodilating effects: They act by stimulating the release of prostacyclin (a prostaglandin hormone) and a vascular relaxing substance. These chemicals also improve the tone of blood vessels and reduce the stickiness of red blood cells, so that they flow more smoothly through the blood vessels as they carry oxygen throughout the body.

Numerous research studies confirm the benefits of ginkgo extracts on all parts of the circulatory system, including improving blood flow and oxygenation to the brain, heart, and other vital organs and the extremities.

It is useful for many conditions including coronary artery disease, peripheral vascular disease, cerebral vascular insufficiency, diseases of the eye due to diabetes mellitus or poor circulation, Alzheimer's disease, Reynaud's disease (vasoconstriction of the extremities), impotence due to diminished blood flow, cyclic edema due to PMS, and even clinical depression (gingko acts as a potent mood elevator).

Many important performance traits are enhanced by the improvement in the oxygenation of the body that occurs when using ginkgo. These include improvements in physical energy, mental clarity, cognitive function, mood, and ability to socialize. Side effects are rare; however, women should be aware that the flavonoid quercetin, which is found in ginkgo, may lower estrogen production within the body. This can be beneficial, however, in women who are in premenopause and are suffering from conditions related to estrogen dominance like PMS and fibroid tumors

Suggested Dosage: Only standardized extracts should be used (standardized to 24 percent flavonoid glycosides and 6 percent terpene lactones). Dosages may vary between 40 to 60 mg, two to three times a day.

Gotu Kola

Gotu kola (Centella asiatica), also called centella, has been used since prehistoric times in India. It has been used both internally and externally, based on its ability to heal wounds and treat skin conditions such as eczema, varicose ulcers, and leprosy.

In the 1880s, gotu kola was incorporated into the French pharmacopoeia. (American consumers sometimes confuse gotu kola and its rejuvenating activity with kola nuts, which are stimulating because they contain caffeine.) Gotu kola has an action similar to Siberian ginseng, acting as a potent anti-fatigue nutrient. People who experience excessive levels of anxiety may find the energy-supporting qualities of gotu kola quite helpful.

Gotu kola was used in China to delay senility. Its effectiveness in improving mental function is beginning to be confirmed by modern studies. It has been used to increase the mental abilities of disabled children. The primary active components of gotu kola are triterpene compounds. These are asiatic acid, madecassic acid, asiaticoside, and madecassoside. These triterpenes liberate the neurotransmitter acetylcholine, which is important for cognitive function. And it is assumed that because of this, mental capacity often improves. Gotu kola also has a tranquilizing effect and counteracts stress.

Suggested Dosage: If using a standardized extract, take 60 to 120 mg per day. If taking the crude dried plant leaves, take 2 to 4 g per day.

Mucuna Bean

The tiny mucuna bean has also been shown to increase your libido and restore your sex drive. This power-packed legume can be traced as far back as Medieval times, and was first described in the English literature in 1804. While every part of the plant is full of medicinal promise, the greatest bene-fits come from the seeds and root.

The key to mucuna's reputation lies in its rich store of L-dopa, one of the few natural sources of the precursor to dopamine, your brain's neurotransmitter responsible for energy, alertness, and libido.

Dopamine is normally made from the amino acids phenylalanine and tyrosine, which must be taken in through your diet and then converted to dopamine within your nervous system. Up until age 45, levels of dopamine remain fairly stable in your body. However, after 45, levels decrease by about 13 percent every 10 years.

The aphrodisiac qualities of mucuna have been known for centuries. In fact, it is one of two primary treatments for low libido in India. An animal study from the journal *Fitoterapia* confirmed this benefit. Researchers found that the mucuna bean can produce "striking improvement in normal mating behavior, potency, and libido and substantiates its use as a sexual function improver."

Another exciting area of research for mucuna involves Parkinson's disease, which is often char-acterized by symptoms such as muscular rigidity, resting tremor, slowness of voluntary movement, and difficulties with balance and walking. In the early 1920's, it was discovered that when dopamine levels were abnormally low, sym-ptoms associated with Parkinson's appeared.

As a chemical messenger between nerve cells, dopamine helps sensory and motor neurons communicate, thereby regulating motor coordination, muscle movement, etc. Without dopamine, these messages are not passed between the nerve cells, thereby resulting in Parkinson's disease.

Due to its high concentrations of L-dopa, researchers looked to the mucuna bean for a possible answer to this disease. In 1995, scientists gave a derivative of the mucuna bean (HP-200) to 60 Parkinson's patients for 12 weeks. Initial dosages were 7.5 grams of the herb derivative in powder form, mixed with water, and administered orally three times a day. The dosage was then increased at the second and fourth weeks. By the end of the study, the average daily dose was 45 grams of HP-200. At that time, researchers found that there was statistically significant improvement in the patients' conditions. The only adverse effects included nausea and vomiting in a few patients.

Suggested Dosage. If you would like to try mucuna to put the pep back in your sex life, I recommend taking 300 mg/day in capsule form, standardized to 60 mg L-dopa.

Note: If you are currently taking antidepressant medications such as Zoloft or Prozac, you should check with your physician before using mucuna.

10

Herbs With Estrogen-Like Effects

Many herbs have estrogen-like activity, including black cohosh and red clover, as well as many others. These herbs have been used medicinally as part of traditional healing practices and have recently begun to be evaluated through research studies. Many of them are very helpful in reducing symptoms due to estrogen deficiency such as seen in menopause. While their estrogenic activity is a small fraction of the activity of the estrogen a woman produces (at least 400 times less active), their benefit is that these herbs cause no or few unwanted side effects, unlike conventional HRT. The use of these herbs has become increasingly widespread with women's growing concerns about the dangerous side-effects of HRT.

Black Cohosh

One of the most effective of the estrogen-like herbs is black cohosh. Native to America, black cohosh was well known and accepted in Native American herbal medicine and was widely prescribed in colonial times as a treatment for menstrual cramps and menopausal symptoms.

The effectiveness and safety of black cohosh are well documented. Clinical studies have shown that black cohosh reduces PMS symptoms such as mood swings, anxiety, tension, and depression. It also relieves the symptoms of pain and discomfort due to menstrual cramps. Other studies have focused on the symptoms of menopause and have found that black cohosh relieved hot flashes, night sweats, heart palpitations, headaches, and vaginal dryness and atrophy. It is also effective in relieving other symptoms such as depression, anxiety, sleep distur-bances, and a decline in libido. Black cohosh is considered a safe and effective therapy.

Currently, in Germany, a special extract of black cohosh is the most thoroughly studied and widely used natural alternative to hormone replacement therapy. This research has prompted at least six well-publicized studies on the standardized extract of black cohosh and its ability to treat menopausal symptoms. According to a review of five key studies on black cohosh from the American Journal of Medicine, black cohosh is most effective at easing hot flashes.

In one of the largest studies on black cohosh, women with menopausal complaints received 40 drops of liquid black cohosh extract twice a day for six to eight weeks. Within four weeks of treatment, a distinct improvement was seen in nearly 80 percent of the women. After six to eight weeks, all symptoms had completely disappeared in half of the women.

Another study found similar results. Scientists gave women with menopausal symptoms either high- or low-dose black cohosh for a 12-week period. At the conclusion of the study, approximately 80 percent of both patients and physicians rated the treatment as "good to very good." The investigators reported no differences in either effectiveness or adverse reactions between the two groups.

Other studies have focused on black cohosh and its relationship to breast cancer. One in particular concluded that black cohosh actually inhibits the growth rate of breast cancer cells due to the herb's lack of estrogen-like effects in certain breast cancer cell lines whose growth is dependent upon estrogen.

Laboratory experiments have shown that black cohosh inhibits the effects of estrogen induced stimulation and actually binds to those receptors. By doing so, it does not increase production of endometrial cells, nor does it change the makeup of vaginal cells. Also, it does not exert estrogen-like effects on the endometrium or breast, nor does it exhibit any toxic, mutagenic, or carcinogenic properties.

Given its apparent safety, I consider black cohosh a safe therapy for women who suffer from the acute symptoms of menopause, such as hot flashes, night sweats, sleeplessness, vaginal dryness and mood swings. I am particularly fond of Klimadynon from BioNorica. Compelling research from several different journals, including *Maturitas: The European Menopause Journal* and *Menopause: The Journal of the North American Menopause Society* has shown that Klimadynon (CR BNO 1055) safely and effectively eases hot flashes and night sweats, promotes plumping of the vaginal wall, decreases vaginal dryness, and even promoted bone growth. Moreover, Klimadynon did not cause proliferation of the uterine lining or of breast cells. This means that it, very likely, does not increase your risk of uterine or breast cancer.

I think that it is important to mention, however, that a recent study from the *Australian Adverse Drug Reactions Bulletin* found that, in rare instances, black cohosh can cause liver toxicity. More common and minor effects include occasional gastrointestinal disturbances, headaches, heaviness in the legs, and possible weight problems. There are no known drug interactions and the only contraindication is in pregnancy, with the possibility of premature birth due to overdose.

Additionally, an article in the *Journal of Agricultural & Food Chemistry* found that some three of 11 tested black cohosh supplements didn't even contain the herb! Instead, they contained less expensive extracts of a similar Chinese herb. To be sure this doesn't happen to you, I suggest buying black cohosh from a reputable retailer or look for BioNorica's Klimadynon brand.

Suggested Dosage: To treat your menopausal symptoms safely and effectively, I suggest taking 40–80 mg of a standardized extract of black cohosh such as Klimadynon twice a day. This dose should contain 2 to 4 mg of the active components (triterpenes, calculated as 27-deoxyacteine). You should see results within four weeks. In my practice, I have seen women experience relief from hot flashes and mood swings in as little as two days to one week.

Red Clover

Red clover can be beneficial for easing hot flashes and improving cardiovascular health. Red clover contains four phytoestrogens (estrogen-like plant compounds thought to have an effect on menopause-related symptoms such as hot flashes) called genistein, daidzein, biochanin, and formononetin, and has become increasingly popular among menopausal women here in the United States.

While some studies have questioned the efficacy of red clover, comparing it to that of a placebo, it does appear to help reduce hot flashes. According to a review of five studies published in *The American*

Journal of Medicine, red clover helps to significantly reduce the frequency of hot flashes. Other research has shown that the herb is also beneficial for cardiovascular health. Both the aging process and menopause itself reduce the elasticity of major arteries (called arterial compliance). This tends to make blood vessels more rigid and less flexible. Over time, these changes can lead to high blood pressure, or hypertension, and increase the workload on the heart. In one placebo-controlled study reported in the *Journal of Clinical Endocrinology and Metabolism*, red clover improved arterial compliance. Other known potential cardiovascular benefits of red clover isoflavones include the inhibition of platelet clumping or aggregation, which can clog arteries, and the herb's action as a potent antioxidant, which also helps reduce buildup of "bad" LDL cholesterol in arteries.

Suggested Dosage: If you would like to try red clover, I recommend taking a standardized extract that contains 40 mg of total isoflavones.

Yin Herbs

Traditional Asian medicine maintains that health and well-being are believed to be a balance of two equally important, but opposing, principles — yin and yang. Yin is associated with attributes such as femininity, receptivity, calmness, coolness, and moisture. Yin also regulates the fluids, blood, and tissues of your body, as well as its structural components, including flesh, tendons, and bones. Yang, on the other hand, is associated with masculinity, aggression, heat, and dryness. It also regulates your body's energy, which acts as the spark plug to your structural elements.

Balance between yin and yang is essential if you are to achieve and maintain optimal health and well-being. In younger, healthy women, the balance between this duality seems to be maintained almost effortlessly. Young women can become either very yin or very yang in response to the demands and stresses in their lives. They can study hard, work overtime, eat anything they want, and still have the ability to return to the balanced middle point, where yin and yang co-exist as a unified reality.

Maintaining an optimal yin-yang balance becomes much more difficult once you reach middle age and menopause, when it's common to experience symptoms such as hot flashes, night sweats, tissue dryness, insomnia, mood swings, and thinning of skin, hair, bones, and connective tissue. In the traditional Asian medical model, these symptoms occur, in part, because yin becomes deficient.

To help bring your body back into balance, I suggest using a variety of yin herbs that work on the kidney network to improve blood and fluid circulation, ovarian health, and your sleep-wake cycle. In particular, I'd like to focus on royal jelly, dong quai, and saffron.

Royal Jelly

Royal jelly—the food of the queen bee—has been used for centuries to promote reproductive health and longevity and ease menopausal symptoms. Doctors from France have reported that women who ate royal jelly during menopause had a complete remission of symptoms, and some were even able to conceive again! Other doctors have found that royal jelly had a libido-increasing effect and helped promote vaginal secretions. Additionally, royal jelly has been found to be a natural antibiotic, fat metabolizer, immune booster, and metabolic catalyst, and even supports adrenal health.

Suggested Dosage: I recommend using ¼ teaspoon of the liquid form of organic royal jelly twice a day. Royal jelly can be purchased at most health food stores. Recent reports have shown that royal jelly imported from China has been found to contain trace amounts of a dangerous antibiotic called chloramphenicol. To avoid this concern, be sure to purchase royal jelly that is produced by bees from the United States under healthy, organic conditions. In addition, women who are allergic to bees or have asthma should not take royal jelly.

Dong quai (also called dang gui)

This Chinese herb has been used for thousands of years as a female health tonic and to prevent or treat symptoms of PMS and menopause. Traditionally, dong quai has been used to treat abnormal menstruation and menopausal hot flashes. Many naturopathic physicians and herbalists today regularly prescribe this herb for their female patients. In China, most women consume dong quai as a food, cooking the root in soup or other liquid mixture to soften it.

Suggested Dosage: I recommend that you take dong quai in powdered form in a 500 mg capsule. Take two capsules two to three times a day. Do not take dong quai is you are on a blood-thinner, as it may reinforce the effect of the anticoagulants and could increase your risk for bleeding.

Saffron

Saffron is a bright yellow Indian spice that is derived from the flower of the crocus sativus. Each saffron crocus grows to be 8 to 12 inches high and bears up to four brightly colored flowers. The dried stigmas of the flowers make up the spice saffron that is used both as a coloring and flavoring agent in cuisines in many parts of the world. It is one of the costliest herbs by weight and is very labor intensive to gather.

Saffron is also revered for its medicinal properties. It is used to reduce menopausal symptoms, enhance calmness, and reduce irritability. To preserve its medicinal properties, stir saffron into hot, cooked food.

Suggested Dosage: Use 1/10 of a teaspoon or less per day, as higher amounts can be toxic, causing stomach and intestinal maladies, and even death. In addition, too much saffron can have a narcotic effect, causing sedation and sleepiness.

Formula D-34

I also want to tell you about an amazing multi-herb blend called Formula D-34. This impressive blend of 10 herbs also works to restore kidney yin. In fact, a study of 20 menopausal women found that Formula D-34 significantly increased blood levels of estradiol, the most potent and chemically active estrogen produced by your body. Additionally, the women reported a considerable reduction in menopausal symptoms, including hot flashes, depression, and anxiety. Formula D-34 is made by Draco Natural Products.

11

Herbs Which Help to Promote Progesterone Production or Balance Estrogen and Progesterone

A number of herbs have been shown to support the production of progesterone. This is very beneficial for women who have health issues related to estrogen dominance. These include PMS, fibroids tumors of the uterus, benign breast disease, endometriosis, heavy and irregular menstrual bleeding and other conditions. These herbs can be a very useful addition to dietary and nutritional supplement programs to help bring women into better hormonal balance during the premenopause and perimenopause transition. I have found them to be very helpful for many of my patients.

Maca

Maca — referred to as either Lepidium peruvianum or Lepidium meyenii — is one of the most traditionally used and valued Peruvian herbs, due in large part to its rich nutrient concentration.

This malty, butterscotch-flavored root contains a number of minerals, vitamins, fatty acids, plant sterols, amino acids, and alkaloids, among other phytonutrients.

In terms of minerals, calcium makes up 10 percent of maca's mineral content. Significant amounts of magnesium, phosphorus, and potassium are also present in this herb. Maca also contains a number of vitamins and amino acids, including B1, B2, B12, vitamin C, vitamin E, and quercetin, as well as arginine, lysine, tryptophan, tyrosine, and phenylalanine.

German and American researchers begin studying Peruvian botanicals in the 1960's and 1980's. They quickly discovered that maca has many health benefits, including relieving menopausal symptoms; stimulating and regulating the endocrine system (adrenals, thyroid, ovaries, and testes); increasing energy, stamina, and endurance; regulating and normalizing menstrual cycles; and balancing hormone levels.

Maca appears to act as a central nervous system stimulant, at the level of the hypothalamus and pituitary gland. It works to stimulate hormone production, which is a critical part of regulating a woman's physiology. It also operates as an adaptogenic herb to help regulate hormones produced by the endocrine glands. It does this by stimulating your ovaries and adrenals to produce the hormones you need; in the levels you need them.

This was shown in a study published in the *Journal of Veterinary Medical Science*. Researchers tested the effects of maca on mouse sex hormones. They found that while progesterone and testosterone levels increased significantly in the mice that received the maca, their estradiol levels were not increased. In other words, the maca helped to raise the levels of progesterone and testosterone to offset the blood levels of estradiol in the mice. Clinical experiences with conditions like fibroid tumors which are triggered by estrogen dominance appear to support these findings although more human research still remains to be done. This is potentially exciting news for women suffering from estrogen dominance.

Suggested Dosage: A traditional dosage of maca is 2-10 grams a day. However, dosages are unique to each woman, so you will need to determine which dosage works for you. There have been no acute toxic effects of maca, even at very high doses. In fact, many Peruvians eat it every day!

Note: I suggest beginning at the low end of the recommended dosage, as too much can cause headaches, breast tenderness, or hot flashes. If you are sensitive or allergic to herbs, you may want to use maca cautiously. It is recommended that you avoid maca if you have a hormone-related cancer (due to lack of formal studies), liver disease, if you are pregnant or nursing, or if you are currently taking conventional HRT.

Licorice Root

Licorice root has been used medicinally for several thousand years in both Eastern and Western cultures. Prescribed for problems including respiratory infections, peptic ulcers, abdominal pain, and malaria, licorice is especially useful in treating PMS, which can be caused by a dominance of estrogen in relation to progesterone levels.

A review article published in the *American Journal of Natural Medicine* indicated that licorice root can lower estrogen while at the same time raising progesterone. Licorice promotes an increase in progesterone by inhibiting the enzyme necessary for its breakdown. Licorice root is also a phytoestrogen. The potency of licorice root is 400 times weaker than estradiol, the most potent form of estrogen created within the body.

Licorice is also useful in counteracting the common PMS symptoms of bloating and breast tenderness caused by water retention. Licorice blocks aldosterone, the adrenal hormone that limits the excretion of sodium, and as sodium attracts fluids, aldosterone can cause fluid retention (edema).

Suggested Dosage: To treat PMS symptoms, a woman should take licorice beginning on the fourteenth day of her cycle until menstruation begins. Licorice can be taken as a fluid extract in a 1 milliliter dosage, one to three times per day. One ml is equal to one full dropperful of the herb in a 1 oz. bottle.

It can also be taken in powdered form in a 400 or 500 mg capsule. The dosage is one to two capsules one to three times per day. Licorice is not recommended for individuals with a history of kidney failure or hypertension, or who are currently taking medic-ations made from digitalis.

Chaste Tree Berry (Vitex agnus castus.)

The chaste tree that yields these berries is native to the Mediterranean. As the name suggests, chaste tree berries were used in traditional botanical medicine to dampen libido. The berries have a unique effect on hormone function. The hypothalamus and pituitary glands in the brain help regulate hormone pro-duction, and chaste tree berry has a profound effect on these two glands. It increases the production of luteinizing hormone (LH). LH is the pituitary hormone that triggers ovulation at midcycle, thereby promoting the production of progesterone during the second half of the menstrual cycle.

Chaste tree berry also inhibits the release of follicle-stimulating hormone (FSH). FSH is needed to stimulate estrogen production during the first half of the menstrual cycle. The end result is to promote the estrogen-to-progesterone ratio in favor of progesterone.

Consequently, chaste tree berry can help normalize the secretion of hormones and bring estrogen and progesterone levels into a healthful balance. This makes it a useful treatment for conditions related to estrogen excess, such as PMS and perimenopause.

Suggested Dosage: The dosage for chaste tree berry is 20 mg of the standardized extract, taken twice a day, in the early morning and evening. It is also manufactured as a 10:1 extract. If taken as a liquid, a typical dose is 1 ml once or twice a day. One milliliter is equal to one full dropperful of the herb in a 1 oz. bottle. It may take a while for the benefits of chaste tree berry to manifest, typically about three months or so.

Dandelion root

To maintain a balance of estrogen and progesterone and prevent symptoms of PMS or premenopause, it is important to support the liver in its function of breaking down and excreting hormones. The liver must produce sufficient bile, which then passes through the gallbladder and into the intestine. In traditional Chinese medicine, when this action of the liver is sluggish, the liver is said to be congested. Herbalists treat PMS with certain herbs to stimulate bile production and thereby bring hormones back into balance. Dandelion root, as well as fennel seed and milk thistle, are commonly used to support liver health.

Suggested Dosage: Dandelion is available in 500 mg capsules. Take one to three capsules three times per day.

12

Herbs with Testosterone-Like Effects

Neurotransmitters are naturally occurring chemicals that relay electrical messages between nerve cells throughout your body, but especially your brain. Research studies have shown that neurotransmitter production within the brain is particularly important for the production of sex hormones, including testosterone. Testosterone is the hormone that has been linked to sex drive, assertiveness, strong and thick bones and tissues as well as energy and zest for life in women

Particularly important for testosterone production are the excitatory neurotransmitters, namely epine-phrine, dopamine, and norephinephrine, have powerful antidepressant effects. They also support arousal, alertness, optimism, zest for life, and sex drive. This additionally supports the beneficial effects of testosterone on your body.

The amino acids phenylalanine and tyrosine are precursors for these excitatory neurotransmitters. Phenylalanine is an essential amino acid that must be taken in through the diet, while tyrosine is produced from phenylalanine. Without proper levels of these nutrients, your dopamine, norephinephrine, and epinephrine levels will most likely be decreased. This can lead to low libido, depression, and other conditions also associated with low testosterone levels.

A number of herbs support the production of testosterone, the excitatory neurotransmitters within the brain or have testosterone-like effects within the body.

Ginkgo Biloba

The Ginkgo biloba tree originated about 250 million years ago, and a single tree can live as long as 1,000 years. It is often planted in urban settings, lining fashionable streets and decorating parks, as it resists disease, insects, and pollution.

Modern science is finding that this ancient plant has a wide range of benefits, including improving blood flow, preventing the brain from aging, and improving all four stages of sexual response—desire, excitement (lubrication), orgasm, and resolution. These are powerful testosterone like effects on sexual function. It has even been shown to reverse sexual dysfunction in women taking certain antidepressants.

When it comes to helping improve blood flow, there is no debate as to ginkgo's benefits. Three hundred published scientific papers and 40 double-blind studies have proven its efficacy. This is due, in large part, to the rich store of antioxidant bioflavonoids found in ginkgo. This also allows this amazing herb to help improve circulation and fight inflammation in just about every organ system in the body, as well as scavenge free radicals.

As for your brain health, ginkgo increases blood flow and energy production, as well as improves production of neurotransmitters; chemicals that help transmit nerve signals. Plus, ginkgo protects brain and nerve cells from deteriorating by stabilizing cell walls and scavenging free radicals that can destroy delicate cell structures. It also helps maintain the brain's supply of energy in the form of glucose and oxygen. This is beneficial, as it supports healthy neurotransmitter- and brain-based hormone prod-uction.

Suggested Dosage: I suggest taking 30 mg of Ginkgo biloba extract (standardized to 24 percent flavonoid glycosides and 6 percent terpene lactones) three times a day. Ginkgo is extremely safe and side effects are uncommon.

Mucuna Bean

Like phenylalanine and tyrosine, the tiny mucuna bean has also been shown to increase your libido and restore your sex drive. This power-packed legume can be traced as far back as Medieval times, and was first described in the English literature in 1804. While every part of the plant is full of medicinal promise, the greatest benefits come from the seeds and root.

The key to mucuna's reputation lies in its rich store of L-dopa, one of the few natural sources of the precursor to dopamine, your brain's neurotransmitter responsible for energy, alertness, and libido.

As I indicated above, dopamine is normally made from the amino acids phenylalanine and tyrosine. Up until age 45, levels of dopamine remain fairly stable in your body. However, after 45, levels decrease by about 13 percent every 10 years.

The aphrodisiac qualities of mucuna have been known for centuries. In fact, it is one of two primary treatments for low libido in India. An animal study from the journal *Fitoterapia* confirmed this benefit. Researchers found that the mucuna bean can produce "striking improvement in normal mating behavior, potency, and libido and substantiates its use as a sexual function improver."

Suggested Dosage. If you would like to try mucuna to put the pep back in your sex life, I recommend taking 300 mg/day in capsule form, standardized to 60 mg L-dopa.

Note: If you are currently taking antidepressant medications such as Zoloft or Prozac, you should check with your physician before using mucuna.

Tribulus Terrestris

This is a weedy, flowering plant native to warm temperate and tropical climates, such as those found in southern Europe and Asia, northern Australia, and Africa. Also known as cat's head, devil's thorn or devil's weed, puncture weed, Maltese cross, and Mexican or Texas sandbur, tribulus is most commonly used for its ability to boost testosterone levels by raising LH and GnRH levels.

GnRH stimulates the production of LH, which stimulates the production of the androgenic hormones, including testosterone. By increasing GnRH and LH levels, tribulus allows you to enjoy the benefits of optimum testosterone levels (such as strong muscles and a healthy sex drive), without the risks associated with excess testosterone).

According to several studies, tribulus is highly effective in increasing both fertility and libido. One animal study found that tribulus increased sexual response in castrated rats. The rats experienced both increased mounting behavior, as well as greater blood flow to the penis. This benefit has also been seen in humans. Research has shown that women taking tribulus enjoyed both increased libido and enhanced emotional well-being.

Suggested Dosage: To enhance testosterone production and increase libido, I suggest taking 100 - 200 mg of tribulus terrestris per day.

Maca

Maca — also known as Lepidium peruvianum or Lepidium meyenii — is one of the most traditionally used and valued Peruvian herbs. At one time, this malty, butterscotch flavored root was considered so valuable that the Incas limited its use to their royal court.

In the 1960's and 1980's, German and American researchers begin studying Peruvian botanicals, and were captivated with what they discovered. Due to its incredibly high nutrient content, maca soon became known as "the lost crop of the Andes."

Specifically, maca contains a number of minerals, vitamins, fatty acids, plant sterols, amino acids, and alkaloids, among other phytonutrients.

In terms of minerals, calcium makes up 10 percent of maca's mineral content. Magnesium, phosphorus, and potassium are also present in significant amounts. It contains smaller amounts of iron, silica, iodine, manganese, zinc, copper, and sodium. Maca also contains a number of vitamins and amino acids, including B1, B2, B12, vitamin C, vitamin E, and quercetin, as well as arginine, lysine, tryptophan, tyrosine, and phenylalanine.

Maca has been used for decades (if not centuries) to stimulate and regulate the endocrine system (adrenals, thyroid, ovaries, and testes); increase fertility; enhance libido; and increase energy, stamina, and endurance. However, it is most commonly known for its ability to increase sexual desire.

According to a research study published in *Andrologia*, maca does improve sexual desire. In a double-blind, placebo-controlled study, researchers looked at different doses of maca as compared to placebo to determine if maca had an effect on sexual desire. They found that maca improved sexual desire within eight weeks of treatment, and that the desire was still present at 12 weeks.

Unlike that Viagra, which works at a circulatory level, maca works at the hormonal level. That's why maca's use isn't limited to men. It has also been shown to improve sexual activity and satisfaction in women by increasing vaginal lubrication.

Maca can also be used to balance hormone levels. As an adaptogenic herb, maca can help to regulate hormones produced by glands in the endocrine system. Unlike conventional hormone replacement therapy (HRT) and even phytoestrogens, all of which work to mimic your body's hormones, maca helps your body produce its own unique balance of hormones. It does this by encouraging your ovaries and adrenals to produce the hormones you need, in the levels you need them, apparently more toward the progesterone and testosterone side of the equation.

This was shown in a study from the *Journal of Veterinary Medical Science*. Researchers tested the effects of maca on mouse sex hormones. They found that while progesterone and testosterone levels increased significantly in those mice that received the maca, their estradiol levels were not increased. In other words, the maca helped to raise the levels of progesterone and testosterone to offset the blood levels of estradiol.

Suggested Dosage: A traditional dosage is 2-10 grams; however, dosages are unique to each woman, so you will need to determine which dosage works for you. There have been no acute toxic effects of maca, even at very high doses. In fact, many Peruvians eat it every day!

Note: If you are naturally sensitive or allergic to herbs, you may want to avoid maca altogether, or at least use it cautiously. In any event, I suggest starting with the low end of the recommended dosage, as too much can cause increased hot flashes, breast tenderness, or headache. It is also recommended that you avoid maca if you have a hormone-related cancer (due to lack of formal studies), liver disease, if you are pregnant or nursing, or if you are currently taking conventional HRT.

Spice Up Your Sex Life

Researchers have shown that certain scents have particularly strong aphrodisiac-like qualities, especially cinnamon, cloves, ginger, and nutmeg. In addition to using these spices when cooking, place potpourri or essential oils that include these scents in your bedroom, bathroom, or wherever the mood strikes you.

Keep in mind that these herbs support the yang in Chinese medicine. They are heating and drying. Therefore, if you are having hot flashes, vaginal dryness due to menopause, you should not use these herbs. Conversely, if you are bloated, carry excess weight, and need to "contract," then these spices may be very beneficial unless you have a specific intolerance to one of them.

Cinnamon — When the Crusaders returned to Western Europe from the Far East, they brought a reputed sexual stimulant with them — cinnamon. Today, this spice is one of the most common herbs across the globe.

Cloves — The Persians, Egyptians, Europeans, and Arabians all considered this spicy scent to be an aromatic aphrodisiac. In the Sudan, women concoct a wedding potion that consists of clove mixed with musk, cherry, and sandalwood. They then wear the blend to the party so its aroma will drift in the air as they dance the night away.

Ginger — The ancient Persian physician Avicenna used to mix this fragrant spice with honey as a cure for impotence. Whether its benefits are due to its pungent aroma or its ability to increase circulation, ginger soon grew to be known as the spice of "burning desire' Today, women in Senegal wear ginger in their belts in order to attract men, while female New Guineans can't say no to a man who emits ginger's strong scent.

Nutmeg — While this spice has a strong smell, it is actually a relaxing scent that relieves anxiety and stress, and even reduces blood pressure. The Chinese are particularly fond of nutmeg's aphrodisiac qualities.

They have found that it can elicit a feeling of rapture and invigoration. In North America in the 1700's, men and women often added nutmeg to their nightcaps. Maybe our ancestors were onto something!

13

General Endocrine Gland, Energy Support and Anti-Aging

Adaptogenic herbs support the adrenals, ovaries, testicles, thyroid and other endocrine glands, thereby preventing the long-term adrenal burnout and exhaustion that occurs with chronic stress. (An adaptogen is a substance that is able to safely increase resistance to a wide range of adverse physical, chemical, and biochemical factors, and promotes a normalization between extremes.) These herbs also contain a wide variety of chemicals that help the body recover more quickly from hard physical labor, athletic exertion, and even convalescence from surgery.

Panax Ginseng

Panax ginseng is an ivy-like ground cover originating in the wild, damp woodlands of northern China and Korea. Its use in Chinese herbal medicine dates back more than 4000 years. In colonial North America, ginseng was a major export product. The wild form is now rare, but panax ginseng is a widely cultivated plant.

Ginseng has a legendary status among herbs. While extravagant claims have been made about its many uses, scientific research has yielded inconsistent results in verifying its therapeutic properties. However, enough good research does exist to demonstrate ginseng's activity, especially when high-quality extracts, standardized for active components, are used.

Ginseng has a balancing, tonic effect on the systems and organs of the body involved in the stress response. It contains at least thirteen different saponins, a class of chemicals found in many plants, especially legumes, which take their name from their ability to form a soap-like froth when shaken with water. These compounds (triterpene glycosides) are the most pharmaceutically active constituents of ginseng. Saponins benefit cardiovascular function, immunity, hormone production, and the central nervous system.

During times of stress, ginseng acts as a general stimulant, delaying the alarm phase in Selye's classic model of stress. The saponins in the ginseng act on the hypothalamus and pituitary glands, increasing the release of adrenocorticotrophin, or ACTH (a hormone produced by the pituitary that promotes the manufacture and secretion of adrenal hormones). As a result, ginseng increases the release of adrenal cortisone and other adrenal hormones, and prevents their depletion from stress. Other substances associated with the pituitary are also released, such as endorphins. Ginseng is used to prevent adrenal atrophy, which can be a side effect of cortisone drug treatment.

In a double-blind study published in *Drugs Under Experimental and Clinical Research*, two groups of volunteers suffering from fatigue due to physical or mental stress were given nutritional supplementation over a twelve-week period. One hundred sixty-three volunteers were given a multivitamin and multi-mineral complex, and 338 volunteers received the same product plus a standardized Chinese ginseng extract. Once a month, the volunteers were asked to fill out a questionnaire during a scheduled visit with a physician. This questionnaire contained eleven questions that asked them to describe their current level of perceived physical energy, stamina, sense of well-being, libido, and quality of sleep.

While both groups experienced similar improvement in their quality of life by the second visit, the group using the ginseng extract almost doubled their improvement, based on their questionnaire responses, by the third and fourth visits. Thus, gin-seng, when added to a multivitamin and multi-mineral complex, appears to improve many parameters of well-being in individuals experiencing significant physical and emotional stress.

Many of my patients have used ginseng and have found it to have energizing effects, especially Korean red ginseng, which is considered to be hotter (more "yang") and stronger than other forms of ginseng, including Chinese and American, which are more cooling (more "yin") and calming in their effects. While Korean ginseng is well suited to men, women may find the effects of this form of ginseng too extreme for the female body.

Some women experience extremely heightened levels of libido with the use of Korean ginseng, as well as tremendous surges of energy. However, it can also disrupt the menstrual cycle, causing a decrease in normal menstrual flow and dryness of the skin and mucous membranes. As a result, women tend to do better with Chinese or American ginseng.

There is evidence in animal and human studies that ginseng increases stamina and endurance. Studies show that ginseng prevents fatigue, lengthening the time it takes to reach exhaustion. Ginseng also enhances mental capacity, as demonstrated in both animal studies and clinical trials in humans. Improvements in logical deduction, reaction time, mental arithmetic, alertness, and accuracy have been observed. ACTH (the hormone that stimulates the adrenal cortex) and adrenal hormones, which ginseng stimulates, are known to bind to brain tissue, increasing mental activity during stress.

Suggested Dosage: For maximum benefit, take a high-quality preparation, an extract of the main root of a plant that is six to eight years old, standardized for ginsenoside content and ratio. Companies manufacturing ginseng products may mention the age of the plants used in their products as a testimony to their products' quality. Take a 100 mg capsule twice a day. If this is too stimulating, especially before bedtime, take the second dose midafternoon, or take only the morning dose.

Siberian Ginseng

Siberian ginseng (Eleutherococcus senticosus) belongs to the same family as panax ginseng, but the exact composition differs considerably. The most pharmacologically active constituents in Siberian ginseng are eleutherosides, some of which are similar in structure to the saponins contained in Asian ginseng. Siberian ginseng has been used in Asia for nearly 2000 years to combat fatigue and increase endurance. The medicinal properties of this plant have been studied in Russia, with a number of clinical and experimental studies demonstrating that eleutherosides are adaptogenic, increasing resistance to stress and fatigue.

According to a review of clinical trials of more than 2100 healthy human subjects, ranging in age from nineteen to seventy-two, published in *Economic Medicinal Plant Research*, Siberian ginseng reduces activation of the adrenal cortex in response to stress, an action useful in the alarm stage of the fight-or-flight response. It also helps lower blood pressure.

In this same study, data indicated that the eleutherosides increased the subjects' ability to withstand adverse physical conditions including heat, noise, motion, an increase in workload, and exercise. There was also improved quality of work under stressful work conditions and improved athletic performance. Siberian ginseng can be of benefit to athletes and also to a person working hard to meet a deadline. Ginseng may help a person push beyond their normal capacity when the only way to finish a job is to pull an all-nighter. Herbalists have also long prescribed Siberian ginseng for chronic-fatigue syndrome.

One way in which ginseng may increase energy reserves is through its ability to facilitate the conversion of fat into energy, in both intense and moderate physical activity, sparing carbohydrates and postponing the point at which a runner, for instance, may "hit the wall." This occurs when stored glucose is depleted and can no longer serve as a source of energy. Siberian ginseng is also used to treat an assortment of psychological disturbances, including insomnia, hypochondriasis, and various neuroses. The reason ginseng is effective may be its ability to balance stress hormones and neuro-transmitters such as epinephrine, serotonin, and dopamine.

Suggested Dosage: Siberian ginseng has virtually no toxicity, although individuals with fever, hypertonic crisis, or myocardial infarction are advised not to use it. A standard dosage of the fluid extract (33 percent ethanol) ranges from 2.0 to 4.0 ml, one to three times a day, for periods of up to sixty consecutive days. An equivalent dosage of dry powdered extract concentrated at a ratio of 20:1 is 100 to 200 mg. Take in multiple-dose regimens with two to three weeks between courses.

I have had a number of patients over the years who have bought inexpensive ginseng, either as a root or in capsule form, expecting miraculous results, given ginseng's venerable reputation. Unfortunately, these cheaper grades of ginseng rarely, if ever, deliver the punch that individuals expect—that is, the chemical equivalent of an auxiliary set of adrenal glands, testicles, or ovaries.

I have, however, seen some remarkable results with high-grade ginseng purchased from reputable Chinese pharmacists that sell top-of-the-line herbs or American companies selling herbs of equivalent quality. Given that the potency of the therapeutic chemicals takes many years to develop within the ginseng root, it is no surprise that, with ginseng, you get what you pay for. Individuals with a serious interest in using ginseng for its adaptogenic properties should search out the reputable dealers.

Licorice Root

Licorice has been enjoyed over the centuries as a candy, but it is also an herb with medicinal properties, featured in the great recorded herbals for 4000 years. Respected by the ancient Egyptians, licorice was among the treasured items archaeologists discovered (in great quantities) when they opened King Tut's tomb. Sometime around the year 1600, John Josselyn of Boston listed licorice as one of the "precious herbs" brought from England to colonial America.

Licorice is used to treat respiratory conditions, urinary and kidney problems, fatty liver, hepatitis, the inflammation of arthritis, and ulcers. The herb also exhibits hormone like activity. Licorice root increases the half-life of cortisol (the adrenal stress hormone), inhibiting the breakdown of adrenal hormones by the liver. As a result, licorice is useful in reversing low cortisol conditions and helping the adrenal glands rest and restore function.

Licorice also contains potent estrogen like chemicals. Since estrogen has profound mood-elevating effects, licorice has antidepressant properties. For a person under a lot of stresses, licorice may be the needed antidote because of its energizing and antidepressant actions.

Suggested Dosage: A standard dosage is 1 to 2 g of powdered root administered at three separate times per day. Licorice has activity similar to aldosterone, the adrenal hormone responsible for regulating water and electrolytes within the body. As a result, taking large doses of licorice (10 to 14 g of the crude herb) can lead to high blood pressure, water retention, and sodium and potassium imbalances.

Licorice should not be taken by children under age two. Caution should be used with older children, pregnant and nursing women, and people over sixty-five. Start with low dosages and increase the strength only if necessary.

Gotu Kola

Gotu kola (Centella asiatica), also called centella, has been used since prehistoric times in India. It has been used both internally and externally, based on its ability to heal wounds and treat skin conditions such as eczema, varicose ulcers, and leprosy. In the 1880s, gotu kola was incorporated into the French pharmacopoeia. (American consumers sometimes confuse gotu kola and its rejuvenating activity with kola nuts, which are stimulating because they contain caffeine.) Gotu kola has an action similar to Siberian ginseng, acting as a potent anti-fatigue nutrient. People who are experiencing excessive levels of anxiety may find the energy-supporting qualities of gotu kola quite helpful.

Gotu kola was used in China to delay senility. Its effectiveness in improving mental function is starting to be confirmed in modern studies. It has been used to increase the mental abilities of disabled children. The primary active components of gotu kola are triterpene compounds. These are asiatic acid, madecassic acid, asiaticoside, and madecassoside. These triterpenes liberate the neurotransmitter acetylcholine, which is important for cognitive function. And it is assumed that because of this, mental capacity often improves. Gotu kola also has a tranquilizing effect and counteracts stress.

Suggested Dosage: If using a standardized extract, take 60 to 120 mg per day. If taking the crude dried plant leaves, take 2 to 4 g per day.

14

Mood-Balancing and Sleep Promoting Herbs

There are a number of mood-balancing herbs that calm and relax the nervous system. The herbs described below have a notable relaxant effect and help to promote a sense of peace, calm and well-being. This is particularly beneficial in women who are feeling stressed and upset. Many of these herbs are also beneficial for women who suffer from insomnia and sleeplessness.

Kava Root

The kava plant is native to the Pacific Islands and is a member of the black pepper family. It thrives in warm, moist climates, where it grows abundantly, reaching a height of fifteen to eighteen feet. As a medicinal plant, herbal preparations are made from the root. It has been used for centuries during social and tribal ceremonies to encourage a greater sense of well-being and relaxation. Pacific Islanders also used kava to relieve pain and enhance mental clarity.

Modern research has identified kava lactones, or pyrones, as the active ingredients in the plant that are most responsible for its potent antianxiety and sedative effects. Kava root contains between 3 and 9 percent kava lactones. European extracts of kava are standardized to contain as much as 70 percent kava lactones for medicinal use.

Kava is used to reduce pain (when first swallowed, it produces a numbing sensation within the mouth). It is also used to reduce anxiety and relax tense muscles. One small study even found it to be useful in controlling epileptic seizures.

Suggested Dosage: The standard dosage is 140 to 210 mg of the herbal extract of kava lactones per day to reduce anxiety and nervous tension. Kava should be taken with meals. It may also be taken before bedtime for the treatment of insomnia. It should not be used for more than four- to eight-week periods without consulting your health care practitioner.

A Caution on Using Kava: As with prescription antianxiety medications, kava may cause drowsiness. Individuals experiencing this side effect should avoid driving while using kava. It may also cause mild intestinal symptoms in some individuals. Rarely, kava has been known to cause a yellowing of the skin or a skin rash. Kava should be avoided by pregnant and lactating women. Finally, kava should not be used with other medications that affect the central nervous system, such as barbiturates, antidepressants, and alcohol or even other sedative herbs like valerian root.

St. John's Wort

St. John's wort has been used for centuries in Europe as a remedy for lung, kidney, and skin conditions as well as a treatment for depression. It also grows in the United States, particularly in northern California and southern Oregon.

St. John's wort is currently much in vogue as a natural antidepressant and has been researched for its mood-elevating effects. Its most important active ingredient is hypericin, which is thought to have antidepressant and antiviral effects. Other substances contained in St. John's wort, such as flavonoids and xanthones, are also thought to have antidepressant effects, thereby increasing the efficacy of the herb for the treatment of depression.

Suggested Dosage: Extracts of St. John's wort are normally standardized to 0.3 percent hypericin. This should be taken three times daily, with meals. Herbal tinctures of St. John's wort may also be used in dosages of 1 to 2 ml, three times a day.

A Caution on Using St. John's wort: Do not use St. John's wort with prescription antidepressants. Pregnant or lactating women should also avoid its use. St. John's wort has few side effects, but it may make the skin more light-sensitive. Individuals using St. John's wort may therefore need to avoid exposure to strong sunlight.

Valerian Root

Valerian is a perennial plant widely distributed in the temperate regions of North America, Europe, and Asia. It is most often cultivated for medicinal purposes. The dried root has a distinctive odor now thought offensive, but in the sixteenth century, it was considered fragrant and laid among clothes as a perfume. In World War I, valerian was used to prevent frontline troops from developing shell shock, and in World War II, it was used to reduce anxiety among civilians exposed to air raids.

Valerian is listed in the French, German, and Swiss pharmacopoeias as a sedative and is traditionally used for relief from insomnia, hysteria, fatigue, intestinal cramps, and other nervous conditions. In herbal terms, valerian is a calmative (a sedative, or depressant), a carminative (good for upset stomach and digestion), a nervine (a tranquilizer), and an anodyne (a pain reliever). The volatile oils are perhaps the most active components.

Valerian is especially beneficial because it normalizes the autonomic nervous system, acting as a sedative when a person is agitated and as a stimulant in the case of fatigue. It balances the opposing forces, the parasympathetic and sympathetic aspects of the nervous system, helping to maintain homeostasis.

While some sedatives may relax a person to the extent that reading a report or cooking dinner becomes an uphill struggle, valerian is known to actually increase concentration, reasoning powers, energy levels, and motor coordination. Herbalists recommend valerian for childhood behavior disorders and learning disabilities. There are no hypnotic or depressive side effects when taking appropriate amounts of valerian, and no morning sleepiness.

The therapeutic effects of valerian are well documented in scientific literature. In a study appearing in the *Journal of Medicinal Plant Research*, volunteers received either a placebo or 450 or 900 mg of an aqueous extract of valerian root. The time it took volunteers to fall asleep was shorter with valerian than the placebo, but the higher dosage of valerian produced no further improvement.

In another study, published in *Pharmacology, Biochemistry and Behavior*, 128 people rated their quality of sleep, taking either a placebo, a valerian extract, or an over-the-counter valerian preparation. With valerian, individuals subjectively reported shorter sleep latency (the time they lie in bed before falling sleep) and a significant improvement in sleep quality, especially among people who considered themselves poor or irregular sleepers.

Suggested Dosage: Because valerian has an unpleasant taste, it is more palatable in capsule form. The standardized extract of valerian (0.8 percent valeric acid content) is preferred to other forms, taken as a mild sedative. The standard dosage is 150 to 300 mg, taken thirty to forty-five minutes before retiring. Valerian is generally regarded as safe and is approved for food use by the FDA.

Individuals who tend to have dryness of their tissues, such as menopausal women, may not like the drying effect that valerian root can have. Rather than abandoning the use of a natural sleeping aid altogether, try melatonin or 5-hydroxytryptophan instead. If one type of therapeutic agent doesn't work, another often will.

Passionflower

Spanish explorers discovered passionflower in Peru, where it was highly prized as an herb by the mountain people. The flower was introduced to Europe and eventually brought to North America by colonial settlers. Passionflower is considered a mild sedative or nervine that reduces nervous tension, anxiety, and blood pressure and also encourages deep, restful sleep, free from frequent wakening. Because it can allay general restlessness, it is recommended for schoolchildren who have difficulty concentrating.

Passionflower sedates the central nervous system due to the presence of small amounts of harmala alkaloids. This herb also has a particular effect on serotonin, a substance produced in the brain that promotes sleep. Passionflower maintains body levels of serotonin by inhibiting the breakdown or metabolism of the serotonin already present. The enzyme monoamine oxidase (MAO) normally converts serotonin to an acid. The class of medications known as MAO-inhibitors keeps this from happening, as does this MAO-active herb. An MAO-inhibitor can double the serotonin content of the brain in less than an hour, and even though passionflower is only a mild MAO-inhibitor, it can still have considerable effect.

Suggested Dosage: Use 1 tsp. of dried leaves per one cup of boiling water to make tea. Let steep ten to fifteen minutes. For insomnia, drink a cup of tea before bed. Three cups a day may be taken for other uses. Passionflower is generally considered safe, but because the harmala compounds are uterine stimulants, it is suggested that pregnant women not use the herb.

Skullcap

Skullcap is a blue-helmeted flowering plant. It is traditionally used as a tonic for nervous tension and insomnia. Herbalists consider it one of the best nerve tonics ever discovered. It acts through the cerebrospinal centers, and its active components are its bitter principles and a volatile oil, scutellarin. Skullcap is used for insomnia, exhaustion, and lockjaw.

Suggested Dosage: To take as a tea, pour one cup of boiling water onto 1 to 2 tsp. of dried herb and let infuse for ten to fifteen minutes. Drink once a day, or as needed. To be of benefit, skullcap needs to be taken regularly for a long period of time. Take one to two capsules before bedtime for its sedative effect.

15

Relaxant and Antispasmodic Herbs

Many people with anxiety suffer from the unpleasant physical symptoms of tight, tense muscles in vulnerable areas of their bodies (the neck, shoulders, jaw, and upper and lower back are common areas to store tension). The following relaxant herbs help to relieve the muscle tension and spasm that often accompany stress. These are also often effective in relieving stress-related indigestion and intestinal gas.

Peppermint

Peppermint is a natural hybrid of the two mints, garden spearmint and water mint. Both peppermint and spearmint are used in herbal healing and have similar effects, but peppermint is somewhat tastier and more potent. Especially because it is a digestive, peppermint tea is enjoyed at the end of a meal, diffusing like alcohol and warming the entire body.

The medicinal component of peppermint is a volatile oil. There are more than forty compounds in the oil; menthol, flavonoids, tocopherols, carotenes, and choline are just some of the substances that contribute to its therapeutic effect.

Peppermint has been used traditionally to cleanse and strengthen the entire system, including the nerves. A bath containing peppermint oil is said to be calming. Peppermint also has an antispasmodic effect on smooth muscle. Calcium in muscle cells causes the muscles to contract. Peppermint blocks this influx, which might explain why peppermint has relaxant properties. Peppermint is a suitable treatment for upset stomach and intestinal spasm. As a stomach sedative, it also helps relieve gas.

In a study appearing in *Phytomedicine*, thirty patients (twelve female and eighteen male) received the herbal drug Lomatol, containing peppermint leaves, while sixteen males and fourteen females received metoclopramide hydrochloride drops. Each patient was instructed to take twenty-five drops of the preparation in water twenty minutes before each meal, three times a day for two weeks. By the seventh day, gastrospasms were eliminated in nearly 90 percent of the patients using Lomatol, compared with only 50 percent of the patients on the hydrochloride compound.

Suggested Dosage: Peppermint is commonly taken as a tea, prepared with 1 to 2 tsp. of the dried leaves per one cup of water. Be sure to use the organic dried leaves that are available in bulk or organic leaves prepackaged in tea bags.

Peppermint oil and menthol, when applied topically, can cause contact dermatitis in sensitive persons. Pregnant women are advised to use peppermint only in diluted, beverage-tea concentrations, not potent medicinal infusions. Moreover, the use of peppermint during pregnancy is discouraged for women with a history of miscarriage.

Chamomile

Chamomile is a time-honored herb, called "ground apple" by the ancient Greeks because of its pleasant apple-like scent. Chamomile was used as a stewing herb during the Middle Ages, and today it is enjoyed as a tea by both adults and children throughout Europe and Latin America.

Used medicinally as a relaxant, chamomile calms nerves and promotes sleep, a benefit documented scientifically since the 1950s. The active principles of chamomile include flavonoids, glycosides, and essential oils.

As a relaxant, chamomile depresses the central nervous system, reducing anxiety while not disrupting normal performance or function. Chamomile seems an ideal herb to have on hand, given the demands and pace of modern life. Anyone who is overwhelmed by the demands of running a house-hold while also conducting a business from home might benefit from a chamomile tea break. A calming drink, rather than a cup of coffee, can sometimes better restore clear thinking and the ability to work efficiently. A cup of chamomile can also temper a child's restlessness.

Chamomile also acts as an antispasmodic, helping to relax muscles that can automatically tighten when the fight-or-flight response is activated. As a tonic, chamomile can help prevent stress-related stomach cramps, poor digestion, and irritable-bowel syndrome.

Suggested Dosage: There are two types of chamomile, German (or Hungarian) and Roman (or English), both of which produce the same effects. To take as a tea, make an infusion of 2 to 3 heaping tsp. of chamomile flowers per one cup of boiling water. Let steep for ten to twenty minutes. Drink up to three cups a day. Children under the age of two may be given a weaker infusion. For a chamomile bath, tie a bunch of chamomile flowers into a cloth hung from the tub faucet, and run the bath water through it.

Ginger Root

Ginger has thick, underground stems (tuberous rhizomes), and it is these knotted and branched rhizomes, commonly called the "root," which are used in cooking and for medicinal purposes. Records of its use in China date to the fourth century BC. As an antispasmodic, ginger is effective in relieving the nausea and vomiting associated with motion sickness and morning sickness in pregnancy. The most pharmacologically active compounds in ginger are the various "pungent" principles, aromatic ketones known collectively as gingerols.

As for its effects on stress management, the gingerroot helps stabilize blood sugar levels, preventing the mood swings that erratic highs and lows of blood glucose can trigger. Ginger also increases the efficiency of the digestive processes and thereby the availability of essential nutrients needed for proper maintenance of blood glucose.

Suggested Dosage: Mix ½ tsp. ground ginger or 1 to 2 tsp. grated fresh ginger with 1 tsp. honey. Add one cup of boiling water to make a cup of ginger tea.

16

Herbal Aromatherapy

These essential oils of plants may be used to counteract stress and support health and wellness, an aspect of herbal medicine called aromatherapy. Essential oils are the subtle, volatile liquids that are distilled from a wide variety of plant material, including flowers, shrubs, trees, roots, and seeds. These essential oils of plants may be used to counteract stress and support health and wellness, an aspect of herbal medicine called aromatherapy. I love using essential oils. Many of them have beautiful scents and feel wonderful when rubbed into the skin.

Essential oils are known to contain trace elements of vitamins, minerals, enzymes, hormones, and substances with immunity-stimulating properties. However, much of the therapeutic effect of the oils is due to the specific chemistry of their aromatic compounds. Essential oils are also effective because of their ease of absorption, due to the small size of the molecules that make up the oils.

Essential oils may enter the body in one of two ways. The oils may be absorbed by inhaling the volatile, aromatic compounds through the olfactory system (hence the term aromatherapy), using vaporizers, steam inhalation, or a tissue dampened with a drop of oil that is held to the nose.

When essential oils are inhaled, the aroma of the oil stimulates the olfactory bulb. The olfactory bulb is part of the limbic system, the section of the brain that controls stress levels as well as heart rate, blood pressure, and breathing, all of which can be affected by stress. A whiff of a particular essential oil alters the neurochemistry of the brain and can produce physiological or psychological changes, often in a few seconds.

Essential oils can also be absorbed through the skin via massage. Oils absorbed through the skin travel through the circulatory system and act on the adrenal glands and the thyroid, interacting with various branches of the nervous system.

Aromatherapy has long been used throughout Europe, where its practitioners have developed time-tested applications for certain essential oils. To calm emotions, Victorian ladies routinely sniffed a handkerchief daubed with oil of lavender.

Now, according to a research study, scientists have found that lavender increases the alpha brain waves associated with relaxation. Studies also confirm lavender's ability to induce restful sleep. In a study published in *The Lancet*, researchers took nursing home patients off of sedating drugs for two weeks. They then infused the room with lavender oil. Three patients who had been taking sleeping medications had difficulty sleeping during the two weeks off medication, but with the infused lavender oil they slept as well as with the medication. A fourth patient, who had not been using a sleep medication, reported sleeping better with the lavender oil.

Other essential oils used to reduce nervous tension, fatigue, or mental stress include Roman chamomile, orange, tangerine, lemon, rose, spruce, and ylang-ylang, as well as the culinary flavorings spearmint, marjoram, and fennel. Jasmine, which is an energizing essence, and nutmeg are used in cases of nervous exhaustion, when the stress response is weak.

These tonics can be diffused in the air or rubbed on the wrists, solar plexus, temples, or soles of the feet. Oils such as lavender can be added to bath water or sprayed on bed linens.

Essential oils can be purchased in health food and beauty stores, and by mail order; however, the quality may vary. For the best-quality distillations, look for essential oils packaged in small dark blue or brown bottles. Prices within a particular product line will vary, as some essential oils are far more expensive than others. A product line with similar pricing throughout may be offering oils of inferior quality. Essential oils, provided they are used in the right quantities, are harmless; however, they can be toxic if taken orally.

About Susan Richards, M.D.

Dr. Susan Richards is one of the foremost authorities in the fields of family medicine and alternative medicine. Dr. Richards has successfully treated many thousands of patients emphasizing alternative health and integrative medicine in her clinical practice. Her mission is to provide her patients with safe and effective alternative therapies to greatly enhance their health and well-being.

A graduate of Northwestern University Feinberg School of Medicine, she has served on the clinical faculty of Stanford University School of Medicine and taught in their Division of Family and Community Medicine.

Her Facebook page, Dr. Susan's Healthy Living, has over one million followers. She is also an ordained minister and her ministry receives over a million prayer requests for healing each year.

Notes

Notes

Notes

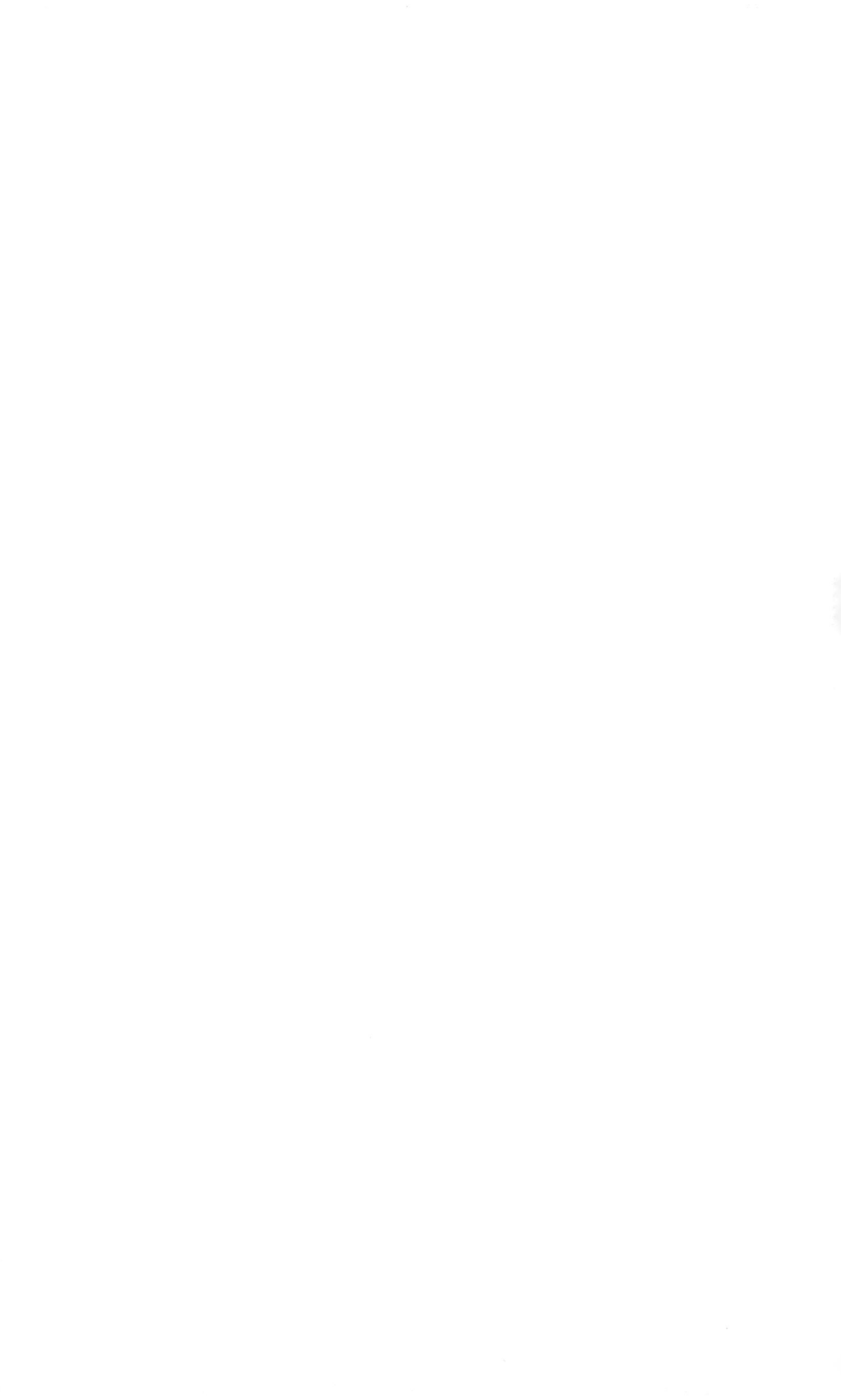

www.ingramcontent.com/pod-product-compliance
Lightning Source LLC
Chambersburg PA
CBHW070919290526
45795CB00001B/361